BARRON'S PARENTING KEYS

KEYS TO DEALING WITH STUTTERING

Patricia M. Treiber

D1056260

BARRON'S

Cover photo by Comstock, Inc. 1993

The information in this book is intended to provide general information, and is presented with the caveat that the publisher and author are not engaged in rendering medical services. If such services are required, a qualified professional should be consulted. The publisher and author disclaim any personal liability for advice or information presented herein.

All inquiries should be addressed to:
Barron's Educational Series, Inc.
250 Wireless Boulevard
Hauppauge, NY 11788
Library of Congress Catalog Card No. 93-3036
International Standard Book No. 0-8120-4666-8
Library of Congress Cataloging-in-Publication Data
Treiber, Patricia M.
Keys to dealing with stuttering / Patricia M. Treiber.
p. cm. — (Barron's parenting keys)
Includes bibiliographical references and index.
ISBN 0-8120-4666-8
1. Stuttering in children—Popular works. I. Title.
II. Series.
RJ496.S8T74 1993
649'.15142—dc20   93-3036
                                      CIP

PRINTED IN THE UNITED STATES OF AMERICA
3456 5500 987654321

DEDICATION

This book is dedicated to my family who support-
ed me throughout the endeavor, to my friends for
their encouragement, and to all the children and
adults who have generously shared their experiences with me, enabling me to learn and grow.

CONTENTS

INTRODUCTION

S tuttering is a speech disorder that generally begins in childhood and persists through adulthood. Unlike many other speech or voice disorders, stuttering has, in the past, been resistant to correction. Without proper intervention, there can be lasting adverse emotional and psychological effects on the individual, as well as an impact on communication between the individual and others. Parents recognize the importance of early intervention when a problem is detected. Living with the daily struggles and the growing anxiety of the stuttering child can increase our own anxiety as well as our desire to provide immediate assistance to alleviate the difficulty.

In my twenty years of experience with children who stutter, I have repeatedly encountered the same questions from parents and the same problems with children. Each parent feels their situation is unique. Unfortunately, there are few clear, definitive answers for parents during this difficult time.

The primary purpose in writing *Keys to Dealing with Stuttering* is to provide parents with basic information on the development of the speech and language process. To understand the contributing factors to stuttering, one must understand the mechanics of the process in order to see where the breakdown occurs. This enables appropriate troubleshooting and designing remediation techniques as well as eliminating some of the anxiety experienced by both the child and parent.

The second intent is to help parents determine the best course for helping their child. Understanding the resources available as well as the process in selecting qualified help can further reduce parental anxiety and help the child.

The third purpose of writing this book is to assist parents in understanding related behaviors that are present during various stages of the child's life that may also compound the speech problem.

There are many things parents can do to assist their child in becoming fluent. Through a better understanding of the problem, the time parents spend with their child can become productive in improving fluency. Parenting is an exciting experience; however, there are many stresses that are associated with embarking on this adventure. It is the hope that these *Keys* will eliminate some of the anxiety associated with dealing with the child who stutters.

Part One

GENERAL
INFORMATION

Many misconceptions exist about stuttering. An awareness of the process of normal speech and language development forms the basis for understanding the problem of dysfluency. This section presents basic information regarding stuttering, its cause, how to identify if it is a problem, and how children who stutter feel about this speech disorder.

1

FACTS ABOUT
STUTTERING

There are several different words used to describe the behaviors called stuttering—dysfluency, stammering, fluency disorders. Each of these labels is used to describe a behavior that interrupts the smooth rhythm and flow of speech. Fluency is a label given by the listener rather than the speaker. While a fluency problem is detectable by the listener, the presence of a real stuttering problem is identified by the speaker who often describes the disruption in his speech pattern as " uncontrollable events" disrupting the attempt to talk.

Although stuttering is more prevalent in school-age children than in the general population, the highest risk level appears to be between the ages of two and a half and four years. Some studies show that the incidence drops by the ages of five and six. However, this can be misleading. Individuals who stuttered in childhood and reportedly "outgrew their stuttering" are often found to exhibit stuttering behaviors in their later years, especially in times of stress.

The stuttering may take many forms. Sometimes parts of words can be repeated (ta- ta- ta- table, ba- ba- ba- banana); sounds prolonged (mmmmmommy); whole words repeated (why, why, why); phrases repeated (do you, do you, do you, do you want it?); or unnecessary sounds, syllables, words and/or phrases interjected into the sentence (ah, you know, well, like).

The speech disruptions may also be accompanied by other physical or motor behaviors that are inappropriate. These may include eye blinking, lip quivering, jaw shaking, and so on. Muscular tension in other parts of the body may also be noted. Unnecessary movements of the hands and feet such as arm swinging or foot tapping may also be present. These are called *secondary behaviors* or *symptoms*.

When negative emotional and avoidance behaviors become associated with the speech behaviors, the diagnosis of stuttering can be more concretely established. For example, if the individual reports being fearful of speaking situations or changes words to avoid having difficulty, stuttering is most likely present.

Unfortunately, stuttering can persist throughout adulthood. It is found in all cultures and in all parts of the world as well as in all races. Stuttering does not appear to be selective. It can be found in all walks of life from the mentally retarded to the gifted and from the poor to the rich. Many famous people were stutterers—Moses, Winston Churchill, and Marilyn Monroe among them. It is significant to note that stuttering did not hinder their ability to contribute to society and lead productive and fruitful lives.

Statistics on stuttering are provided by groups that study the problem, including the National Institute of Health in Washington, D.C. The incidence is approximately 1 percent of the general population indicating that today approximately 2.25 million people stutter in this country. Some researchers feel that this number merely reflects the number of individuals who are presently exhibiting stuttering behavior. The statistics for individuals who have ever reported having difficulty at one time in their life could be much higher.

There is a significant gender difference in the incidence of stuttering. More males than females stutter with statistics ranging from three to four times as many men than women. Some evidence suggests that the gender difference may be similar at the onset of the problem but that more females may recover during childhood, resulting in an increasing proportion of males who continue to stutter in later years.

There is speculation that stuttering is genetically linked. However, the exact cause of stuttering remains subject to controversy. Until this is clarified, a true understanding of all other factors related to the disorder is difficult.

Stuttering tends to run in families. An early diagnostic indicator to determine if a child is actually a stutterer is whether any other family member stutters or has at some point during their lifetime. This fact is often not readily known by other family members since early experiences with dysfluency may be regarded as a normal developmental phase. For this reason, this valuable diagnostic clue can be missed.

When a problem is suspected, parents should seek guidance from their pediatrician as well as from other trained professionals. It is important to seek help as early as possible to avoid the potential anxiety in the child that can develop during the process of learning to speak.

Years ago, parents were told to ignore stuttering behavior in their young children because they would "outgrow it." Today, early evaluation and intervention are more widely accepted and encouraged by professionals in the fields of speech and medicine. This is primarily because speech and language growth and development occur rapidly in the young child. Developing a fluent speech pattern during this time is important to prevent frustration and encourage the ability to interact and communicate verbally. The disruptions in speaking caused by stuttering can interfere with this process and have long-term negative consequences.

2

NORMAL SPEECH DEVELOPMENT

S tages of speech and language development are all approximations based on averages obtained from observing many children. The times given for each level in the following discussion may vary significantly among individuals. Differences are even evidenced among siblings within the same family. Infants born prematurely may show further delays in the completion of each stage. When observing the child, be careful to note only significant variations from these timelines. It is only when there is a major difference that concern is warranted.

Speech starts with the cry at birth. Until cooing begins between two and three months of age, crying is the major form of expression for the infant. Cooing is produced in response to speech. Various sounds are made and may include the first vowel sounds. At approximately four to seven months of age, the stage of babbling begins. During this time, the infant continues to play with sounds and combines many different sounds together. It is an extremely pleasurable time for the infant. Various new noises are produced as the feeling and sensation of movement in the mouth becomes more and more familiar. These vocalizations are heard when the infant is dry, cheerful, well fed and the noises can be increased by social reinforcement—tickling, smiling, or physical contact.

As infants become more aware of the environment, they begin to echo the sounds they hear around them.

These sounds gradually connect into words at approximately one year (although this time may vary). At this point, the infant's gestures, sounds, and noises express a variety of meaning to the parent. Desires and ideas are communicated by combining isolated and meaningless sound units. One of the most memorable moments is when the baby calls for "Da-Da" or "Ma-Ma" for the first time.

Environmental exploration expands with the infant's increased mobility and motor development. The child's first words express numerous different concepts and are primarily the names of toys, animals, food items, and events of the day (bath and potty). Single words expand gradually to two at eighteen to twenty-four months of age, then to three, and soon to more to make the child's intentions and desires more precise. At first, the word *cookie* conveys a variety of meanings as a statement, a desire, or a need. As more words are added and the length of the verbal message increases, the child's communication becomes increasingly more clear and exact ("want cookie," "chocolate cookie," and so on). The child steps away from his parents into the vast world of ideas and communication.

Sentences generally appear at thirty to thirty-six months of age. New nouns, verbs, adjectives, adverbs as well as all of the other essential elements of the language appear almost daily and magically seem to fall appropriately into the child's growing verbal repertoire. Shortly, two and three sentences are common. Often, sentences a paragraph long are the only way the child can contain all of the ideas and discoveries of his expanding horizons!

The growth and development of a child proceeds on many levels that are interrelated yet distinct. Physically, as bones and muscles grow and strengthen, greater mobility is possible. Increases in this strength permit more precise and intricate movement—from crawling to walking and from holding objects with a whole hand to picking up things with tiny fingers.

The art of speaking builds on the growing refinement of these motor skills. Speech requires rapid and intricate movements of the tongue, lips, and teeth. In addition, delicate timing of the muscles for breathing and for sound production only can be accomplished when the physical system has developed and matured to such a state to make this possible.

Cooing, babbling, combining of sounds into words, and, finally, the connecting of words into phrases and sentences is a natural process that unfolds gradually. Although the speaking process is sequential and systematic in its development, the length of each of these steps is unique for each person and anticipated by parents with excitement.

As babies grow physically and their speech progresses, their ability to learn from their environment and put together thoughts and ideas progresses, too. Infants begin to be able to merge what is seen with words that are heard and develop an understanding and idea of things in the world. These ideas create images in children's minds that are reinforced by the environment forming the basis for knowledge and communication. These are called concepts.

It is important to note that although each of these processes—physical development and communication— are interrelated, their complexity often requires the total attention and concentration of the growing child. Growth is inconsistent; for example, some motor skills speed ahead whereas others—such as speaking—lag behind. Although the growth process is sequential and must follow in an orderly fashion, there are individual timing variations that occur among the areas of speaking, motor development and thought development, as well as within each area. Ultimately the process evens out and all the pieces fit precisely into the complex puzzle—the child.

3

NORMAL DYSFLUENCIES

M ost normal speakers demonstrate the types of behaviors described as *dysfluency* periodically in their general speaking. Individuals can be heard to repeat words, sounds, and phrases. At times, there are even silent pauses while the speaker tries to determine the word for which he is searching. Speech is often plagued by the addition of unnecessary words or phrases. Many teenagers and adults utilize words such as *like* and *you know* to mark places between thoughts. Experts indicate that probably no one is 100 percent fluent all of the time!

Children who are in the process of learning to talk may also demonstrate these same behaviors. The degree of their dysfluency can vary from day to day. These changes in levels of fluency may be associated with language development, motor growth, as well as factors in the environment. A breakdown in speaking can occur when a child tries to put into words some of the ideas and concepts he has developed from his environment. The selection of the appropriate words and phrases as well as the correct sentence structure are complicated tasks and may serve to create a breakdown in the fluency of speech. As noted earlier, the growth and development of each individual is unique. Some children may never exhibit any dysfluent behavior during their development. Others may pass through several periods of disrupted speech.

Unfortunately, all too often parents have been advised by physicians and friends that repetitive or disruptive speech behaviors are always a normal part of the speech and language developmental process. Because of this, early intervention was not sought in many cases where it may have proven extremely beneficial. Some signs and symptoms can be utilized to determine if the problem is actually stuttering and if professional intervention is advisable. Those will be covered in Key 4. However, if you feel unsure whether the dysfluency is stuttering or not, seeking appropriate advice and counsel is advised. Experts agree that there is no danger of turning a normally dysfluent child into a stutterer if the proper guidance is employed.

The normally dysfluent period usually occurs between two and five years of age. The child often appears to be stalling while gathering thoughts. Parents report that children seem to be competing for attention with others and once that attention is gained, stuttering or speech repetitions are observed while the child seemingly finalizes thoughts. Generally the first word is repeated. Once this is said, the other words seem to follow without difficulty. The periods of dysfluent speech seem to come and go over a period of time. This stage ultimately passes and speech returns to normal.

4

~~~~~~

SYMPTOMS OF STUTTERING

Sometimes there appears to be an almost violent disruption in the natural process of speech development. The words appear stopped. A single sound may be repeated several times before the rest of the word follows, or a word may be repeated over and over again while the rest of the sentence seems to be suspended in mid-air. Often additional sounds or words are included inappropriately.

The parents want to do something—anything—to make speaking easier, such as finishing the sentence. This may be inappropriate, however, because they don't know what the child is really thinking. The natural flow of ideas becomes distorted by breaks and seemingly endless pauses. The parent tries to remain patient hoping the child doesn't sense concern. One wonders if the child is aware of the struggle and how she feels.

The disruptions don't happen all the time. Often days—even weeks—pass and ideas and thoughts flow easily. No problems appear to exist. The sense is that the child has apparently passed through this difficult period and is now fine. Then, as suddenly as the child stopped, the breaks and pauses return and attempts at speaking are marked by repetitions and other struggles such as eye blinking or foot tapping.

When the difficulty returns, it often seems more intense than before and the efforts to communicate are more frustrating. Although it is difficult to be sure, it seems that the child appears to recognize that something is happening. What was easy the day before now has become difficult. More effort is required to speak today than yesterday. Questions begin to arise: What can be done? What should be said to help?

It is sometimes easy to tell when a child has become aware of a speaking difficulty. The following behaviors are some of the early signs:

1. Physical movements such as putting a hand to the mouth or patting the leg or arm when trying to speak in an attempt to help the words come out (secondary behaviors)
2. Increased facial movements (including eye blinking) indicating a struggle and increased forced attempts to speak
3. The consistent insertion of the unnecessary words such as "um, like, so, ah, and"
4. The observable substitution of one word for another, especially when the choice is less appropriate

Less easy to detect are the efforts to avoid struggles in speaking. These include prolonged silence while waiting for the tension to pass; complete avoidance of situations that may be deemed to cause a problem such as speaking to strangers or playing with certain friends; or using nonverbal behavior such as pointing instead of speaking to communicate.

Although the age may vary, dysfluent speech is generally first noticed around the age of two and a half to three years when single words are combined into sentences

13

and the ideas being expressed are more complex. The sentences and verbalizations are longer. The ordering of the words, that is, sentence structure, becomes more complicated. Although this age is frequently identified as the beginning of stuttering for the real stutterer, the age of the child is not the significant factor. Other factors that contribute to the identification of the dysfluency as stuttering include the reaction to the speech disruption by the child, the presence of these other motor or struggle behaviors, and the stress created by the increased length and complexity of the language that she is using.

Factors in the environment and a family history of stuttering also serve to highlight the probable presence of real difficulty. The fact that a family member is a stutterer does not necessarily predict that all future children also will eventually and inevitably become stutterers. But if the child is dysfluent, and other realtives are stutterers, there is increased risk that she will not outgrow the problem.

Age is not the most critical factor in the evidence of stuttering behavior. Thus, the absence of any observable stuttering during the child' s speech and language developmental period does not ensure the absence of future fluency problems. The problem can occur at any time in people's lives if they are predisposed to becoming a stutterer.

A primary factor that differentiates normal dysfluency from stuttering is the amount of the dysfluency. Researchers tend to believe that stutterers generally have twice as many dysfluencies in speech as the normal child. Another factor to consider is the number of repetitions and interjections as well as the type of pattern the child uses when she is dysfluent. Observations of abnormal airflow and the use of the sound *ah* in the repeated syllable tend to be signals of potential future problems. Some authors indicate that stuttering children tend to repeat sounds longer than do nonstuttering children, who may repeat a sound only once or twice.

To summarize, a family history of stuttering, the presence of secondary behaviors, awareness of difficulty, frequent repetitions, and interjections are early signals of a stuttering problem.

5

WHAT CHILDREN SAY ABOUT STUTTERING

W orking with a large number of children of a wide variety of ages helps to provide some insight as to how they regard themselves and their speech difficulty. Although theorists have long encouraged parents to ignore stuttering behavior or dysfluency in young children, experience has shown that most often children are keenly aware of the difficulty they are experiencing, regardless of their age. The mother of a three-year-old reported that her son came to her crying and she asked what had happened to him, because he suddenly was unable to talk. However, the most important information about the emotional effects of stuttering is gleaned from adults who have weathered this storm. These individuals range from those who feel they have outgrown their dysfluency and are now only occasionally dysfluent, to people who still evidence considerable difficulty and continue to seek help.

When struggling through a speech barrier, a secondary physical reaction may be triggered. This can be a source of fear. At first it is uncomfortable. For some children, the speaking process will become painful. As stated earlier, children may choose to speak less and retreat into the more comfortable world of silence, using hands, gestures, and pointing instead of words to communicate.

Most young stutterers know that the attempt to produce sounds and words meets with some type of physical opposition. They realize that they are unable to speak when they want to start to speak. This inability to do what they want when they want can create increasing frustration in the child. New opportunities to speak can then create anxiety with the anticipation of the struggle that may follow. Research psychologists report that the beginning stutterer may feel annoyed, frustrated, helpless, and sometimes embarrassed. The episodic nature of early stuttering may result in these feelings disappearing during periods of fluency, only to return with greater intensity when stuttering recurs. All of these factors serve to heighten stress and tension in the child. This may, in turn, lead to avoiding situations where speaking may be necessary.

Other children confronting the same situation may, however, choose to continue the struggle. For them, this pattern of forcing words will become the norm. They become unaware that they are using any extraordinary physical movements. These behaviors become habits. One child may become fearful and withdrawn, while another shows no apparent negative impact.

When asked if they have difficulty speaking, many young children will indicate that the words "get stuck" when they are trying to say them. Others who may not feel as secure, will outwardly deny that there is any problem but will be noted to avoid doing things that might involve speaking. Young children who stutter will often answer questions with "I don't know" rather than risk potentially getting stuck on what they want to say. This can lead to the impression that the child is "stupid" when he may, in fact, know the answers to simple questions.

Children describe the difficulty as "getting stuck," "the words are blocked," "I can't say what I want to say," "the sounds get stuck," "I keep repeating things over and over and over again." One child stated that he "tumbled over words." While many are unable to indicate where they physically think the problem is occurring, some will say that "their throat gets tight" and the words apparently "get stuck there."

In the early stage, the reaction of others may also have a profound effect on the child's perception of their dysfluency. The anxiety of parents, siblings, grandparents, friends, and strangers about the dysfluent behavior of the stutterer also can create anxiety in the child. If children observe concern from these authority and support sources, then they may also feel anxiety. They sometimes feel that what they are doing must be wrong to evoke such tension. They are unable to control what is happening, which can lead to frustration. Again, some children will exhibit no such negative reaction.

Experts agree that if children are unaware of their speaking difficulties at a young age, this lack of awareness generally does not generally last too long. With few exceptions, if children have not realized the difficulty themselves, children in school will readily bring it to their attention. The insensitivity of youth, as well as some adults, leads to ridicule and mockery of struggling stutterers. Embarrassment and hurt can become associated with speaking. Since there is nothing within their power to control the problem, a sense of helplessness can develop, leading to negative feelings and, eventually, further avoidance behaviors.

The negative emotional components identified that affect the child can include fear, anxiety, apprehension, embarrassment, helplessness, loss of control, doubt, and diminished self-confidence. It is believed that these per-

18

ceptions begin to formulate early in life. The exact timing is unique to each individual and cannot be generalized. The degree to which they are actualized and felt is also highly individualized.

Some adults who stutter describe the unexpected disruption or blockage of normal speech production as feeling as if they are suddenly "possessed." The unpredictability, as well as the unknown source, of the blockage is frightening. Because of this, self-confidence is challenged. A fear of stuttering at an important moment develops. A sense of a loss of control sets in.

To summarize, children are aware of their difficulties in trying to speak. It is often surprising to parents when they ask their children what kind of difficulties they are having. Although the youngest children may not be able to identify the problem, they are quite perceptive and will answer affirmatively when asked if words sometimes get stuck when they are trying to speak. Awareness level may be more obvious for some children, such as the crying child who seeks help from the mother to end the struggle. The important issue is to provide information to help reduce the anxiety and potential fears that can develop from stuttering.

6

~~~~~~

THE CAUSE OF STUTTERING

Developing the ability to speak is considered a science because of its physical basis. Theories explaining the process continue to develop as knowledge of the human body and its intricacy expands. Our scientific understanding of the workings of the human body is incomplete and evolving daily.

The fields of psychology, physiology, and speech-language pathology have all contributed numerous reasons for the causes of stuttering. One clear, definitive explanation does not exist. The broad categories used to define and explain stuttering are *organic* and *environmental*. These theories each illustrate a certain aspect of the problem but do not focus on a completely integrated picture of the stutterer. The fifteenth edition of the *Handbook of Pediatrics* defines stuttering as "a transitory normal phenomenon appearing in some children during periods of distress." The definition goes on to state that when emotional tension is relieved, the stuttering disappears spontaneously. While this offers a basic description, it falls short of offering a clear understanding of what may be causing the problem. There is general agreement among experts that there are multiple causes of stuttering and that an unknown genetic predisposition is suspected, making certain individuals particularly vulnerable. In the following paragraphs, organic or neurophysiological theories and environmental theories are discussed.

Neurophysiological Theories

Neurophysiological theories are based on extensive research by scientists on the speech mechanism and the brain. Current research focuses on the *voice box* (larynx) and its behavior as a source of stuttering. The larynx contains the *vocal cords*—those muscles that are required for speech sound to be produced. Studies have shown that in the stutterer these muscles sometimes become too tense and lock. When an individual in a comfortable situation such as normal speech production encounters an unexpected obstacle—unmoving or locked vocal cords—the automatic response is to struggle and push through the resistance. The reason for the struggle is to achieve the desired normal behavior—vibrating vocal cords. The stutterer makes repeated attempts to return the vocal cords to the effortless, normal movement pattern. This observable struggle is generally what is referred to as stuttering.

Another neurophysiological theory relates the brain to the stuttering process. It is believed that stuttering may be related to faulty structures or functions of the brain. The brain is divided into two parts or hemispheres—right and left. In most normal speakers, the left side of the brain is the origin of speech production whereas the right side is the origin of musical and nonverbal activities. Researchers, utilizing special brain technology (electroencephalography) now can study the electrical activity of the brain. Recordings have suggested that unlike nonstutterers, stutterers process verbal and nonverbal material in the same hemisphere—the right hemisphere. This would make them different from normal speakers and is proposed as a cause for stuttering.

Environmental Theories

Some theorists describe stuttering as variations in speech directly related to changes in environmental stimuli or events. Dysfluency is described as variable depending on the listener. While being able to talk fluently to a child, the same individual may stutter when speaking to an adult. An old theory labeled *diagnosogenic* was accepted for years as the basis of stuttering. This theory stated that it is the parental diagnosis of stuttering that creates in the child the expectation that she is a stutterer rather than her own perception that she has a problem. As a result of, or in response to, the diagnosis, the child believes there is something wrong with her speech and then tries to avoid what the parents have thought is a problem. While popular for many years, this theory is no longer held in high regard.

Theories also exist that define stuttering as a behavior caused by conditioning. It is suggested that children can develop learned avoidance behaviors that become stuttering. This means that because of the parents' negative comments or attempts to correct their child's dysfluency, the child begins to experience anxiety about her own normally dysfluent speech, which eventually makes her fear certain sounds, words, or acts. She then tries to avoid such situations.

Others think that stuttering is a learned behavior that can be reinforced by the events that occur at the time of the stuttering. That is, when an event or behavior occurs, the individual can learn to repeat that behavior based on the way it is received by others. If she is rewarded, then the behavior may occur more frequently. If punishment follows, however, anxiety is created and the behavior tends to be avoided.

In the case of the stutterer, if she experiences dysfluency during a particular situation or event, negative emotions become associated with that particular situation. If the stuttering again occurs in a similar situation, the behavior becomes reinforced. The individual tends to believe that the situation has created the speech dysfluency and she becomes more and more anxious when approaching a similar event. In time, the dysfluent responses may be generalized to other similar situations. The anxiety created serves to increase the stress and, unless the situation can be avoided in the future, will increase the tension with which the individual approaches it. The stuttering behavior becomes paired or learned as part of the situation and not as an event that occurs on its own. Only nonstuttering successes in these similar situations can reduce the anxiety and conditioning related to the event and the speech behavior.

The difficulty with these theories is that there is no functional link between behavior and the speech production process or the physical aspects of stuttering. A more reasonable approach to defining the cause of stuttering would be to combine the aspects of conditioning with those of the physical behaviors of the vocal cords and/or brain.

7

~~~~~~

CHILDREN AND TENSION

E xperts agree that dysfluency in children and adults is aggravated by stress or tension. Tension-provoking situations have a cumulative effect. Many things can make a child or an adult tense. An infinite variety of life's daily events can create a large amount of tension.

The American Psychiatric Association reports that children often have fears that adults don't understand. At certain ages children seem to have more fears than at other ages. Young children often exhibit simple phobias that can be overwhelming fears of specific objects such as animals or situations (e.g., being in the dark). These most often go away without any special treatment. The presence, however, of these fears creates additional stress that is difficult for us to relate to and understand.

Often the commonplace things that are taken for granted can adversely increase tension. Some tension-increasing things include people, authority, excitement, situations, and external events.

People
The addition of another person to a situation can create an increase in muscle tension to anyone else present. The individual does not have to be threatening or even interacting with the stutterer. Interestingly, as the age of that additional person increases in relation to the others, the tension level also increases.

Imagine the daily encounters children may have with others and the mixture of their ages. These can range from their peer level, to older children, to adults. In school, there are daily opportunities to interact on all these levels at the same time. The more people present, the greater the potential increase in tension.

In addition to age, the size and familiarity of the individual also contribute to tension level. Large, powerful people are often viewed as threatening, especially from a child's vantage point! Conversing with strangers can also heighten apprehension. All these reactions are perfectly natural and the degree to which they create tension can vary, although some tension will always be present.

Authority

Another factor that can increase tension level is the perceived authority level or importance of an individual. This may also relate to the age variable that was previously described. It is easy to recall people who are considered intimidating. The obvious ones are policemen, doctors, lawyers, teachers, school principals, and clergy. Other more subtle examples may be relatives, friends, or even someone of the opposite sex.

Think of the effect these people can have on someone who is only 3 feet tall! Communication with them can usually be described, at best, as stressful—even for a confident person. Relief is only felt when the situation has ended and the stressor has departed. Yet the fear and tension may remain for some time afterward. There can remain a lingering stress created by the anticipation that one may have to be with that person again.

Parents are authority figures. They are rule makers, limit setters, and disciplinarians—all attributes of an authority figure. This unavoidably special role can put

25

stress on a child. No one really likes to be corrected, punished, or told what he can and cannot do. Parents often report that their children become more dysfluent around parents whose success at their jobs requires authoritarian and exacting traits. It is often difficult to avoid transferring office conduct to the home environment; children appear to be most sensitive to this.

Excitement

Tension is often associated with negative reactions or situations. However, the muscle tension created by those events is similar to the state created by exciting experiences. Thus, attending a birthday party, playing a video game, or going to a ball game can have the same effect on the body as being called to the principal's office or being the last batter up with two outs and bases loaded!

Situations

Situations that can create stress can be grouped into the *familiar* and *unfamiliar* (or uncertain). Familiarity is created by repetition of the same or similar experiences. These can leave strong impressions, especially if the experiences were negative. These situations are then approached a second time with a level of apprehension or tension. Answering questions in class, striking out at a critical point in a ball game, asking for a date, or playing with certain friends can all create tension if past experiences were not favorable. This tension can be triggered by just the memory of the incident. Tensions can also begin to increase in anticipation of the event, even before it occurs.

New people, places, things, or activities all bring with them a certain apprehension. This is based on an individual's inability to predict whether these things will have a positive or negative effect, or whether they will be beneficial or cause harm. Until this uncertainty is past, they act as

26

stressors. For a child, this is most easily illustrated by the beginning of the school year. From the first day of nursery school or kindergarten, to the beginning of the new grade each fall, apprehension and uncertainty are heightened. Whether anticipated eagerly or reluctantly, the start of the school term is a predictable stressor.

This uncertainty is even evidenced when learning a new skill. To a child, learning to read represents such a situation. The newness of the task, the strangeness of the words, and the insecurity in one's ability to succeed are all tension factors. Adults, for example, experience the same behavior when they read aloud and encounter a new, complicated word. Often, the usually smooth, effortless reading process suddenly becomes disrupted by efforts to navigate this unfamiliar territory.

External events

There are many events that can add stress to the life of a child. Among these can be family arguments, the birth of a sibling, family relocation, and/or divorce of the child's parents, close relatives, or friends. Change of any type brings with it added stress that is felt by the child.

Consequently, either singly or combined, the effect of the above stressors can produce heightened anxiety and tension for the child.

Part Two

~~~~~~

SEEKING HELP FROM TRAINED PROFESSIONALS

O nce a stuttering problem is suspected, the next step is to find the most appropriate help. This section explores the resources available to parents and children to assist in the diagnosis and remediation of stuttering. It then discusses what can be anticipated from the treatment and the child's role in the process. Finally, it offers parents guidance on assisting their child during this time.

8

~~~~~~

WHEN TO BEGIN
SEEKING HELP

When seeking help, parents of very young children who stutter preface their questions to therapists by saying that they are unsure of what to do. They don't know if there really is a stuttering problem or if they are just overreacting. Parents often seek help after an initial period of dysfluency has passed and new stuttering has appeared that is more intense than before. They watch their child struggling and want to do something, but they don't know what. They are usually going against the advice of their pediatrician "to ignore the problem because the child will outgrow it," and seek help at the insistence of their relatives who feel that something is radically wrong.

There are several questions that can help identify if a child is a potential stutterer. These questions summarize the information in Key 6, "The Cause of Stuttering," and provide a quick checklist to determine if the speech difficulty is more than normal dysfluency, signaling that it is time to seek help.

1. Does anyone in the immediate family stutter?
2. Does anyone in the extended family (aunts, uncles, cousins) stutter, or did they at one time and outgrow the problem?
3. Does your child appear to struggle to get words out?

4. Does your child make unnecessary physical movements of any kind such as eye blinking, foot tapping, or hair tugging when trying to say a word?
5. Is your child aware of having difficulty when trying to speak?
6. Does your child appear to be upset or frustrated by the difficulty she is encountering? (For example, does she stop trying to say something once she is stuck? Does she tell you she is having trouble?)
7. Does your child substitute a word(s) rather than say one that she has had trouble with either now or in the past?
8. Does your child get stuck on the first word she is trying to say?
9. Does your child appear to speak rapidly?
10. Did the stuttering appear to go away and then return?
11. Are you, as a parent, anxious, concerned and/or confused about what is happening?

If the answer to any of these questions is yes, then the possibility exists that your child may not be merely experiencing a normal dysfluency stage. Further information about what is happening and what can be done to alleviate the problem would prove beneficial to both you and the child. Simple intervention by the parents at the earliest possible time (for children as young as two or two and a half years of age) can have lasting positive results.

Whatever the age—from two to adult—help should be sought, especially if the stuttering individual expresses concern about her speech. One of the best defenses against future emotional or psychological problems that may arise from stuttering is understanding the cause of the difficulty. This knowledge permits individuals (or their parents) to decide whether they wish to proceed with learning how to manage the problem.

As children grow older (between age 10 and the teenage years), it may not be possible for parents to convince them that help is needed. However, if stuttering first appears at these ages, knowledge of potential causes and methods to control the difficulty prove invaluable to adolescents in making future decisions regarding ways to improve their speech when they feel they are ready.

Therefore, it is never too soon or too late to seek help. At any stage, benefit can be derived for the parent and, especially, the child.

9

SEEKING HELP: THE
PEDIATRICIAN

For most parents, the primary resource person with respect to their child is their pediatrician. The child's physician is usually the primary professional person outside of the family whom they see or consult on a regular basis. Pediatricians are regarded as the specialists in child development.

Unfortunately, advances in the field of speech and language regarding the nature and treatment of stuttering seem slow to be recognized by the medical profession. Experience working in a hospital has shown that the advice given to parents today is no different from that given twenty-five years ago. Most parents are advised by a pediatrician to disregard the early stuttering of their child. The behavior is dismissed as a developmental stage. Parents may be urged to tell their child to slow down when they see a problem, however, the most universally offered advice is *to do nothing and make sure that no attention is called to the problem.* This advice may be based on the theory that recognition of the dysfluency could potentially create real stuttering if the child becomes aware of it.

It is only if dysfluencies persist to the age of four or five years, or when the school system detects a problem, that physicians will advise parents to seek professional help. It is important to note that this is not characteristic of all pediatricians, but it does seem to reflect the advice of a significant number.

There are two problems with this advice. It can potentially have a negative effect on the child by delaying appropriate intervention. This can be evidenced emotionally or with the disrupted development of communication skills. More disturbing can be the effect on the anxiety level of the child. One child who was told that he would "outgrow" the stuttering problem, woke each morning and asked his mom if "today was the day." This question persisted through the age of twelve until additional help was sought and intervention could begin. In another case, a seven-year-old child approached his mother crying when trying to speak and finally asked her "Why can't I talk?"

Parents trust pediatricians and regard them as powerful authority figures. They value their judgment. When parents go against this valued advice, they often view themselves as betraying an important ally and they feel guilty. Each day they see their child struggle, they feel more upset and concerned. However, they are caught between sensing their child suffer and listening to their physician. Seeking additional counsel for further education and understanding of stuttering is often appropriate. It is important to seek outside advice for more in-depth understanding just as one would seek a specialist if a more complicated medical problem arose and better insight was needed.

Once parents have received additional direction, it is beneficial to share this with their child's physician. Parents can serve as an informational source for their pediatricians by keeping them informed of what they have discovered and alerting them to other possibilities for treatment. This will help other children in the future who may be exhibiting the same difficulties.

10

~~~~~~

SEEKING HELP: THE PSYCHOLOGIST

Many people, especially some adult stutterers, believe that stuttering is a psychological problem. Theories discussed in Key 6, "The Cause of Stuttering," reinforced this belief. It is clear that there is a psychological component to stuttering. Those stressors (or stress factors) discussed in Key 7, "Children and Tension," are not always easily identified. Even if they can be, children (and adults) may find it difficult to deal with them. One of the best resources for learning techniques to deal with stress is a psychologist. Many methods exist to help people learn to cope with stress better. In addition, the psychological discomfort associated with stuttering—anxiety and fear— may need to be addressed by a professional if the results achieved through speech therapy do not eliminate them.

Some children exert control over their parents. They sense the anxiety that is present when they stutter, and will use it to their advantage. Others refuse to follow any directives given by their parents. This renders the parent helpless in knowing how to regain or attain control—an important element in being able to help the child learn. Because of this, they cannot successfully assist them. This is rare, but it can happen. These parents (and children) may benefit from talking with a psychologist about how to improve the situation to everyone's mutual advantage.

Some children try to exert control over themselves as well. They can be categorized as high self-stressors. These are people who are perfectionists and become highly upset if they make a mistake. For them, learning new tasks can be very stressful. Because of their impossibly high standards, mistakes are not permitted! Teaching the self-stressor is extremely difficult. In a situation where elimination or control of stress is important—such as the treatment of stuttering—this type of behavior is self-defeating. This behavior can be exhibited by children as young as three or four years of age and can grow increasingly more intense as the individual grows older. Such children may benefit from outside assistance in learning to be less harsh on themselves thereby allowing themselves to become more receptive to learning.

Points to consider in seeking additional counseling include:

1. Does the child seem to be "too hard on herself"?
2. Does the child get upset when she makes a mistake when trying to do a task?
3. Is she a perfectionist in all that she does?
4. Does she refuse to cooperate when an adult tries to teach her something new?

Parents may find speaking to a psychologist helpful for themselves. If they are overwhelmed by their child's stuttering, they may need to seek assistance in exploring their feelings and expectations. It may be helpful to learn how to develop a more realistic and less catastrophic picture of the speech problem. Once parents are given an explanation for the nature of stuttering and understand some of the potential causes, they realize what can be done to control the problem and further help may not be required. The absence of relevant, reliable information about the problem creates anxiety and an unrealistic picture of stuttering which can unnecessarily complicate the situation. (Also see Keys 38, 39, and 40 in Part Five.)

Points to consider for parents considering seeking psychological assistance:

1. Do you have difficulty accepting your child's dysfluencies?
2. Are you overly fearful of the child's future and how it will unfold because of the stuttering behavior?
3. Are you able to work with your child or is there continual conflict when you attempt to give any guidance?

After therapy has begun, additional information has been obtained from a professional in the field of speech-language pathology, and these behaviors persist, further assistance may be necessary.

Experience has shown that older children and adults who have achieved significant success with their stuttering therapy program may reach a plateau that they appear to be unable to move beyond. Occasionally, regression to the stuttering behavior will occur. Despite attempts to re-establish appropriate speech techniques, they will probably feel frustrated as their dysfluency reappears. These individuals may be candidates for counseling. They may need to determine what is hindering their ability to respond to the learning process and discover what is sabotaging their energies and efforts to improve their speech.

Some teenagers (and adults) who were severe stutterers have been unable to use their fluent speech techniques because they were unsure of the reaction of others to their new, fluent self. One individual indicated that he was scared because he knew how people treated him when he stuttered, and, although he didn't like it, he knew what to expect. It was too difficult to cope with the unknown. It was easier to revert to stuttering behavior rather than use fluent speech. In these cases, counseling may also prove valuable.

For the older child and teenager, psychological help may be beneficial if the following questions are answered affirmatively:

1. Have I been in a stuttering therapy program for a long time and have made little progress even though I have applied myself and have had periods of great success?
2. Even though I can use fluent speech, am I fearful of using it in real-life situations?
3. Do I continue to avoid situations because I am fearful that I will stutter?
4. Do I fear how others will react to me when I am using fluent speech? Do I prefer to stutter in most situations and do I feel more comfortable doing so?

In selecting a psychologist, it is helpful to ask if she has experience working with stutterers; how successful she is; what age range she works with; and what techniques she uses. It is also very important that any and all specialists working with the child and/or parent communicate regularly. If the child is seeing a speech pathologist, the psychologist should speak with the parents to coordinate therapy programs. It is most beneficial if the psychologist shares the same belief on the cause or the nature of stuttering and agrees with the treatment being followed. A similar perspective on the therapeutic process can facilitate recovery and be most advantageous to speed the learning process.

11

~~~~~~

SEEKING HELP: THE SPEECH-LANGUAGE PATHOLOGIST

S pecialists trained in the area of communication and its disorders are called speech-language pathologists. They may also be called speech clinicians or speech teachers. They are experts in the field of speech and language development. These individuals all possess a minimum of four years of college training with emphasis in speech pathology. Whereas physicians and psychologists, due to the breadth of their professions, may only devote a small amount of time during their training to the area of communication development, the speech-language pathologist focuses entirely on that subject.

The field of speech and language is broad and encompasses many diverse areas. Language development and disorders, stroke and neurological disorders, speech and sound development and disorders, swallowing and the disorders of swallowing, the care of the voice and disorders of the vocal anatomy are but a few. Each of these areas is a specialty in itself.

Current standards for education in this field require a master's degree level of training. Many states license speech-language pathologists. Therapists must follow strict ethical standards as well as continuing education requirements to ensure that they remain current in their profession to retain their licenses. A majority of professionals in the field also hold credentials from the American Speech-Language-Hearing Association. This credentialing is called the *Certificate of Clinical Competence in Speech Pathology* (CCC-SLP). To obtain this certification, individuals must complete an apprenticeship in the area of speech and language and pass a national examination. Before licensing became a regulation in many states, this certificate was regarded as the most acceptable standard for ensuring the quality and the competence of the professional. Today, the most generally accepted credentials are either a valid state license or the certificate from this association. Many states, however, also offer other credentialing procedures that replace the license or CCC for individuals who are practicing in the public schools.

The following is a list of states. that license their speech-language pathologists:

Alabama	Kansas	Nevada
Arkansas	Kentucky	New Jersey
California	Louisiana	New Hampshire
Connecticut	Maine	New Mexico
Delaware	Maryland	New York
Florida	Massachusetts	North Carolina
Georgia	Minnesota	North Dakota
Hawaii	Mississippi	Ohio
Illinois	Missouri	Oklahoma
Indiana	Montana	Oregon
Iowa	Nebraska	Pennsylvania

Rhode Island	Texas	West Virginia
South Carolina	Utah	Wisconsin
Tennessee	Virginia	Wyoming

All states listed regulate speech-language pathologists through licensure except Minnesota, which regulates through registration.

States and the federal district that do not regulate speech-language pathologists are

Alaska	District of Columbia	South Dakota
Arizona	Idaho	Vermont
Colorado	Michigan	Washington

Courtesy ASHA, March 1993

12

SELECTING A
QUALIFIED SPEECH-
LANGUAGE
PATHOLOGIST

As in psychology, speech-language pathologists are trained in a variety of ways to manage a particular communication problem. The clinician's training program and individual preference dictate the method of the therapy program that will be used. There is no "one right way" to treat stuttering; rather there are a number of possible solutions. In Key 6, "The Cause of Stuttering," the causes of stuttering and theories were discussed. Therapists trained in different theories may focus on different aspects of the problem. Some of the treatment programs have validity and have proven successful. Those that have had the most positive results incorporate a change in speech rate, a reduction in tension level through a systematic and organized approach, and information/education about the nature of stuttering. In addition, because of the different needs of children versus adults, although the theoretical orientation may not change, it is important that the approach to the problem should change when working with different ages.

The selection of a speech-language pathologist should be made as carefully as that in selecting a pediatrician or medical specialist. It is recommended that experience and specialization in the area of childhood stuttering be the primary consideration. The following are questions that can be kept in mind during the selection process:

What is the degree of training of the therapist?

Many states license professionals who provide services to the public. Criteria and procedures are established to ensure the provision of quality care. Professionals are required to meet certain educational requirements, maintain continuing education in their field of expertise, and adhere to codes of ethical practice. A state agency generally monitors the compliance to these standards. If your state requires a license (see page 39), then it is the minimum credential you should accept from a private therapist.

Therapists based in a school may be certified under different standards and by a different credentialing agency. These therapists may not be required to hold a state license. A master's degree in speech-language pathology with undergraduate studies in this field would reflect the most extensive overall training (except for a Ph.D.).

Many therapists are certified by a professional association called the American Speech-Language-Hearing Association. Upon completion of master's level studies in speech, they spend an additional fellowship year in further guided study and must pass a national examination to receive the Certification of Clinical Competence (CCC). In some states, this certificate automatically entitles the therapist to a license. Other states may have additional licensing requirements. School therapists may not be required to hold this certificate.

While degrees and credentials are important indications of educational attainment, some therapists who have been practicing for many years may not have a master's degree but, by virtue of their experience with stutterers, may be even better qualified to provide the best assistance.

How extensive is the therapist's training in stuttering?

Whether the therapist has taken more than one basic course in the subject is important. One college course may be too generalized and does not provide the depth of information necessary to address all the complications that can be associated with stuttering. Supplemental workshops or courses enhance understanding of the problem and provide deeper insight into the intervention process. Whether the therapist seeks further posteducational training should be one of the questions to ask. In addition, how extensive the therapist's experience is in working with stutterers is important to determine. Practical experience is far more valuable than "book learning." Successfully applying what has been learned is a more powerful indication of how helpful they can be in working with the child than a college degree or summary of courses.

How many children has the therapist already treated?

While experience with adult stutterers is indispensable in designing effective treatment for children, working with children who stutter requires different skills. Such experience provides deeper insight into the complications that occur later in life if the problem is not addressed and resolved at a young age. Many therapists are skilled in both areas.

What approach does the therapist use?

There are several successful approaches to the treatment of stuttering. It is important that the therapist be able to discuss the model that she follows and answer any questions regarding its success rate, application, and so on. Parents should feel free to ask the therapist if there are other parents that they may contact to discuss this approach and how it has worked for their children. Requesting references is not inappropriate. Talking with other parents also helps avoid the problems others may have encountered during the course of treatment. These parents can be the best source to give advice on how things really work. Experience has shown that parents are willing to share their insights to help others.

What is the therapist's belief regarding the nature or cause of stuttering?

If the therapist can explain what she perceives or understands to be happening during the stuttering block, she is demonstrating, at least, a basic knowledge and comprehension of the problem. Beware the clinician who says she "doesn't know why, but what she does seems to work." Knowledge and understanding of stuttering are very important for the development of effective treatment strategies. If something in therapy isn't working, the therapist must know what she is doing and why in order to problem solve and develop an alternative approach.

What does an evaluation include?

The evaluation process should be focused on the fluency of the child. Investigate whether the process will involve comprehensive analysis of language structure, sound production, and voice analysis. These elements are not necessarily important when assessing the young stutterer. They are the basic components of a comprehensive assessment of communication skills, but are unnecessary when evaluating fluency.

Other problems in speech and language that may exist in addition to disfluency in the young stutterer are important to acknowledge to determine the primary focus of intervention. If fluency is the primary concern, then energy should be placed on it, with more in-depth evaluation of other communication disorders at a future time.

What is the therapist's goal for the therapy program?

Although "fluency" seems to be the correct response to this question, the answer is more complicated. First, how is fluency measured? If a stutterer substitutes words (as many do), she may appear fluent, but is not. If stress is low, fluency will be improved but the real problem will not be corrected. A better answer would be *utilization of the new speaking technique (whatever the method) a majority of the time, measured by its incorporation into daily life.* The automatic result of use of technique *is* fluency!

The fluency goal of the child (depending on the age) should also be given consideration. In severe stutterers, *improved* speaking capabilities are all that is desired. Motivation to proceed beyond this point is often poor. Fluency all of the time is not important to them. Continuation in therapy beyond this point may not be appropriate. The therapist should be aware of the child's expectations as well as her own. *Technique usage*, not fluency, should be the goal.

Is the parent included in the therapy process? Is the parent present at each therapy session?

Most often the presence of one or both parents is important during the therapy sessions since they play an integral part in the remediation process and should be included in all of its aspects. This promotes better understanding of what is expected at home as well as demonstrating how to work with the child. Sometimes, however, dynamics between parent and child can be disruptive to the therapist's work and may create additional anxiety in the child. If this is the case, then at the very least, a parent should be able to observe the process. Time should also be devoted at the end of each session to have each aspect of the process carefully explained so that the home program can be implemented.

How long are children usually in therapy?

It is not unreasonable to ask how long therapy usually takes. A definitive number of sessions may be difficult for any therapist to predict since learning aptitude is a primary component of treatment and it is often difficult to quantify. Yet, based on past experience, the therapist should be able to offer some estimates on the length of the course of treatment or give direction regarding its process.

What kind of work is required at home?

Practice of the new speaking technique is essential for it to become a habit. Time in therapy is not sufficient to provide the reinforcement needed to habituate the new skill. Therefore, the therapist should be able to indicate what the time commitment will be outside the formal therapy process, as well as outline the type of exercises required. Daily practice is generally the minimum standard. Some therapists think brief, frequent sessions are more appropriate than long periods of practice to maintain interest and motivation. This decision should be based on what is most suitable for the child and her learning style. A rationale for each of the assignments should also be available. It is easier to motivate the child to practice if the goal is understood and a sense of accomplishment can be realized at the end of the session.

Will the therapist work with other specialists (teachers, psychologists, school therapists, etc.) if appropriate?

Integration of new speaking skills into all environments is the ultimate goal of the therapy. The willingness of the therapist to interact with others in the child's world to facilitate this integration will broaden the scope and improve chances for success. Visiting the school, when appropriate, helps not only other professionals but also the child. The child sees a connection between speech therapy and the speaking technique incorporated into a familiar environment. Other professionals begin to understand what stuttering is and how they can help this child as well as others.

Other questions may include:

- How frequently will the therapist see the child?
- Is the therapy "plan" one that can be shared with the parent?
- How is progress measured?
- Will the therapist make home or school visits?
- At what point is outside assistance (psychologists) integrated in the process, if at all?
- Is the type of therapy individual or group therapy?
- Is there a support group to meet and discuss questions and concerns?

These are important issues that should be addressed in the selection of a therapist for a child. Unfortunately, some children have spent many years seeing a therapist once or twice a week with limited improvement in their speech. Parents are often not part of the process and not involved with intervention. Too frequently they wait for a report from the therapist instead of becoming actively involved in their child's treatment. Since the nature of stuttering is more clearly understood today, intervention should prove more successful than in the past or there should be an understanding of why the process is not reaching its desired goals. The answers to the selection questions will help parents to determine to some extent the kind of success that they can anticipate.

13

WHAT TO EXPECT FROM THERAPY

The goal of therapy is to present a new behavior—a speech technique—that is to be learned. It is not to fix a speech pattern that is incorrect but rather to teach a new skill that will be used to replace it. In teaching, it is important to be able to assess if the new skill has, in fact, been internalized or learned. Then it is necessary to see if that new behavior has, in fact, become a habit. These concepts must be incorporated into the therapy process and monitored frequently.

A good therapy program should incorporate these concepts. It is also helpful to the child if the learning process is fun. In treatment programs, the major focus is the teaching of a new speaking technique. This is often supplemented with games to reward the child for the production of the correct speech behaviors and to prevent boredom. It is necessary to determine if the learning task is too demanding and, if so, it should be balanced by an activity that is fun for the child to play. However, with children, there is a fine line between focusing on the concept to be mastered and becoming overwhelmed by the desire to win the game. Careful management of the child during each session is important to stay on course for the desired result to be achieved.

An important characteristic of a good therapist is patience. In all learning situations, patience is an essential virtue for teachers to enable them to adapt to the learning abilities of different students and avoid frustration. Some children are quick to grasp the idea of what behavior is desired. Others may require many repetitions to catch on to the idea. Therapists sometimes abandon a valid treatment program because the child's progress appears too slow. Understanding the learning process and the unique needs of each child requires confidence in the value of the program and patience with the learning process. Patience is vital in being able to maintain a positive and nonstressful environment that is also fun and encourages learning and success.

Flexibility in the therapy process is also valuable. Sometimes the task that is presented may be beyond the grasp of the child. When the therapist is able to modify and change what is required and still achieve the desired result, learning can be facilitated. Sometimes clinicians follow standard programs and are unable to adapt to the individual needs of the child because they are outside the parameters of what has been dictated by the program designers. This methodology can stall progress and prohibit success.

The therapist should be able to present clear goals and be able to measure accomplishment of these goals. Learning is sequential and each stage is built upon the next. This should be explained to the parent as well as the child. Progress should be measurable and continuous based on the goals that are established. A beginning and end to the therapy process should be clearly outlined and each step the child makes toward reaching the goals should be measurable.

Communication should be open and continuous between the therapist and the parents. Parents should always feel that they have the opportunity to ask questions and to clarify their ideas. The therapist should be willing to meet frequently with the parents and, when possible, include them in the therapeutic process.

In addition to all of these elements, a reward system for the child is a valuable adjunct to the therapy program. Learning is accelerated by reward. The idea that learning something new should be reward in itself is admirable. In reality, most of us would not go to work day after day if we were not compensated in some fashion. Enthusiasm can generally be increased if the compensation is also increased. The same applies to the child who is required to learn something new, something that others do not have to spend their time learning—a speech technique. Praise is essential and an important reward in itself. In addition to this, a more tangible compensation such as a toy, ice cream cone, and so on, may also increase the desire to comply with what is requested as well as make the learning process fun.

A final key aspect of a good therapy program is clear home assignments based on the activities of the therapy session. The therapist should set guidelines and goals for the parents with the assignments that address them. A sign of clinical expertise is variability and creativity in the home exercises.

Therapy programs that do not incorporate all of these aspects are not necessarily bad. The most important aspect of therapy is the *outcome*. Steady and significant progress in focusing on improved speaking techniques rather than decreases in fluency are important to consider. Any program that emphasizes the reduction in the frequency of stuttering is not clearly focusing on the appropriate goal.

As discussed earlier, stress is an important component of the dysfluency problem. If stresses are minimal, fluency will be greater. Since most often stress level is hard to track and control, fluency levels can be highly variable based on external factors. Rather than focusing exclusively on fluency, it is important to focus on changing speaking behaviors and assessing how well those new speaking behaviors are learned and habituated. Measuring the amount of incorporation of the new speaking technique into every day situations is a higher measure of therapy effectiveness than any other variable.

The frequency of therapy can be variable. A therapist should be able to give some outline based on the goals and the content of the therapy program as to how often the sessions will be scheduled. Some programs for older children and adults are extensive and may last three weeks with therapy six hours a day. This intensity serves to help establish the new behavior through intensive, constant exercise and drill. Many people respond positively to such a learning approach.

Other therapists vary the frequency of therapy to accommodate the patient's learning style and needs. One approach to consider is that therapy frequency could be tied with continual patient progress. So, if the patient makes great progress for several sessions in a row, therapy sessions could be scheduled further apart. Some therapists may give exercises to be completed at home before the next formal session will be scheduled. Other therapists may see patients more frequently and assist them with the practice of these exercises. It is the individual child's learning style and needs that should dictate how the process is conducted.

It is sometimes valuable to determine the costs of the therapy process prior to selecting the therapist. Some programs bill for the entire process as a complete package.

These costs can range from \$2,500 to \$3,000. Many therapists will bill by the session which may be an hour or a half-hour time period. Parents may call the American Speech-Language-Hearing Association in their state to ascertain a range of costs that would be reasonable in their area. The Department of Consumer Affairs in the state capital should be able to provide this telephone number or other resources to seek.

Insurance coverage for stuttering therapy in the past has been limited. Most insurance carriers cover speech therapy services only for speaking abilities that have been lost due to traumatic events such as accidents or strokes. Calling the benefit specialist of the family insurance carrier prior to beginning therapy is suggested to determine levels of coverage for these services.

14

WHAT TO EXPECT FROM THE CHILD IN THERAPY

P arents sometimes neglect to consider the child's role in the therapy process. The child is often expected to comply with adults' wishes without any discussion or input. Making progress is not always possible with this type of attitude.

As noted earlier, even preschool children may be aware of the difficulty they are encountering when they are trying to speak. One two-and-a-half-year-old boy's favorite "Sesame Street" character was Linda, who was deaf and communicated with sign language. The child, when asked, expressed empathy for her communication disability and her inability to speak that was similar to what he experienced when he was caught in a stuttering block.

A young child exhibits some relief from these anxieties when the difficulty in speaking is acknowledged by the parents. The frequency and intensity of the stuttering has been observed to sometimes automatically decrease once parents communicate with their child that they recognize a problem and are going to seek assistance.

The very young child can learn a new behavior from imitating parents' speech. Because normal speech patterns at this age are newly developed and not as habituated as in an older child, good modeling or demonstrating of the new speaking behavior generally can result in rapid improvement. Praise and encouragement accelerate the learning process of a new behavior.

Parents become frustrated, however, when the child does well in the practice session but goes back to old speech patterns when talking to them. This merely reflects the weakness of the new speech habit and is not a reflection of poor therapy or noncompliant behavior on the part of the child. Parents need to understand this is typical behavior with any age child and should exhibit patience during the learning process.

As the child becomes older, there may be other factors involved besides the change in the speech technique. Not all children are concerned about their dysfluency. For some, it is not considered a problem because their present circumstances do not penalize them for imperfect speech. They have friends who accept them as they are and protect or defend them from others who may not. They may be successful athletes in school or excel in other areas that are socially rewarding; the speech behavior is not an issue. The need to change may not be recognized. Indeed, doing speech homework steals time from other, more high-priority activities such as watching television, playing video games, playing sports with their friends, or talking on the telephone.

Anxious parents, however, can see beyond the present and realize the need to change the speech pattern to avoid future difficulties in school or further into the future—for example, when their child enters the job market. They desire improvement now before there is a penalty exacted because of the stuttering. Unfortunately, children are not as farsighted as this. Their major concern is the present and their feelings at this moment. They do not share their parents' same long-range vision and concern.

All children in elementary school can benefit from treatment even if they fail to see the need. However, the improvement may not be readily evident. The basics of a new, fluent speech pattern can be taught, drilled, and rehearsed, much as in learning to play a musical instrument or a sport. But, just as with the sport or the musical instrument, the child cannot be forced to use them. The learning principles and the understanding will be stored in memory, however, for a time when there is motivation for change. At that point, those principles can be built upon to facilitate further refinement of the skill. Thus, learning a new speaking technique in the therapy situation may evoke immediate improvement in fluency or may not effect a change until years beyond that experience when speaking fluently will be more important.

Intervention is also valuable for older children because, as with the younger child, understanding the nature of the stuttering can reduce anxiety. Older children sometimes become less motivated to work on changing their speech or using their speaking techniques once they understand the principles behind the stuttering. When they know that tension and speed are factors that create stuttering, they feel less anxious realizing that they have a solution to their problem if they should ever need it. They become comfortable enough in their lives at that point to be willing to wait and continue stuttering until a time when they may really need to change. They don't want to be bothered practicing because they have other priorities (play, friends, sports, and so on). Focusing on using the techniques in structured speaking tasks that have immediate reward (such as rehearsing a speech for speech class or reviewing reading material that will be read aloud in class) can sometimes motivate the less interested child.

The adolescent and teenage stutterers are more difficult to help. These young adults are caught between obeying their parents and asserting their own independence. If they begin therapy to please their parents and are not internally motivated to make a change, the process can prove fruitless. An informational session with a therapist to help understand the mechanics of stuttering would be advisable. Although difficult for most parents to accept, the best that they can do at this time is to provide education about the subject and encourage continuation in the therapy process. Most children will seek help when they are ready if they have been exposed to adequate information about what to do and where to go.

One sixth-grade boy best illustrates this. He came regularly to therapy but reportedly did little home practice and continually resisted parental help. The therapist and child decided that a "vacation" from therapy would be advisable since the entire process appeared to be creating more tension—especially between the child and the parent. The mother was not pleased with this decision but agreed. Periodic conversations with the parent over time revealed her continued anxiety about her son's dysfluent speech even though he was doing well in school.

Five years later the boy requested that his mother schedule an appointment to begin therapy again. At this point in his life, he was approaching the college selection process and was concerned about his future. His anxiety was heightened and he was evidently frustrated. He was now highly motivated and immersed himself in what was required to learn the new speaking techniques.

Thus, it is important for parents to consider their child's attitudes as well as their own needs to develop realistic expectations and goals for the child, especially when trying to change the child's speech. The skills can be presented and taught to the child and reinforced by the parent at home, but the child's motivational level and interest in the process must also be considered when looking for success.

15

HOW PARENTS CAN
HELP THE
STUTTERING CHILD

O nce a stuttering problem has been identified, and the
child seems to fit the profile of a stutterer, the parent
becomes an integral part of the change process. At
the earliest signs of stuttering there are some techniques
that can be employed immediately by parents to try to
assist their child.

Some research indicates that diet has a direct effect
upon muscle tension or stress levels. Assess your child's
diet to determine if there may be excessive amounts of
stress elevators present. Seeking nutritional guidance may
be a positive step toward eliminating dietary items that
could elevate muscle tension. Some items may include
caffeine, chocolate, food additives, and sugar. Diet modifications may be employed when appropriate after consultation with a physician or nutritionist. Removal of these
foods for a trial period and observing the child's behavior
can validate if they are adding to the problem.

It is helpful to recognize when your child is experiencing difficulty speaking. Simply acknowledge it. During a
dysfluent time, when your child is evidencing a great deal
of struggling, you can gently tell him you understand that
he seems to be having difficulty. Placing a gentle hand on

his arm or shoulder may also serve to calm and reassure him. If he has been working on a speech technique and he is proficient in its application, you can suggest he try employing it at this time. It is important that the suggestion be made in a supportive manner. Sometimes during these periods of stress, newly learned skills are not easily at your child's disposal and he may not be able to comply. By requesting in a nonthreatening way that he attempt to try his new skill, he may be pleasantly surprised that he is successful. Being understanding and patient at these times is extremely important. Comfort and support during these dysfluent periods can serve to reduce anxiety in your child and may help improve fluency.

During periods when speaking is difficult, speaking to your child in a softer voice and with a slower speaking rate often can reduce some stress and have a soothing effect. This is comforting and calming to the child and can also give him a better model of how to speak than the one that he is using.

For the child who is working with a speech pathologist, the role of the parent becomes more clearly defined. Aside from the previous suggestions, it is essential to monitor and assist the child's speech at home as well as be actively involved in the learning process. Changing an old behavior pattern or speaking technique requires intense practice of the new skill. Most children need support and assistance to achieve the desired outcome.

Children who remain in therapy for years are often those who do not have parental assistance at home. The responsibility for change is left to the therapist (especially in the public schools) to be accomplished in the allotted thirty or sixty minutes each week. Sometimes children are seen only once a week or are included in a group session with no reinforcement of the new skill provided between these sessions. Permanent change and improvement is rare under these circumstances.

Parents need to be actively involved and participate in the therapy process with the therapist. It is recognized that teaching a child a skill requires knowledge on the part of the instructor. Parents do not automatically know what their child needs to learn to improve his speech. Although quick instruction or a review after a therapy session can help, it is usually insufficient to adequately convey the material that should be used at home to learn the assignment for the week. It is beneficial when the parent observes and asks questions throughout the therapy session.

Because stress reduction is an important aspect in stuttering therapy, the conflict created between parent and child during practice can undermine progress. Understanding that practice is essential, parents need to identify how this can be accomplished with the least stress for both parties. Some parents have difficulty working with their own children who may be uncooperative and resistant to practice. Parents in this predicament should find someone—a patient, older sibling, relative, or neighbor—who can work with the child and then do all they can to reinforce the learned behaviors.

Finding time to spend with the child to practice and develop the technique is very important and often difficult for very busy parents. If your schedule does not permit this, again, perhaps someone can be found who is able to follow through and assist with learning on a regular basis. However, this will merely suffice for basic practice time. Parents must be kept aware of what is learned and find opportunities to encourage the use of the new speech technique outside of the practice time. Positive reinforcement through praise for doing the right thing is more meaningful when given by the parent. This is especially important when the use of the new speaking technique is noticed outside of the therapy or practice situations. Parents should never be too busy to fulfill this need!

Parents can often find opportunities to encourage and practice when driving in the car with their child or ordering food in a fast food restaurant. When the child is willing to cooperate and attempts to use his new speech techniques, praise and encouragement from the parent at such a time is highly reinforcing and rewarding for that child. Phrases such as "You sound terrific!" or "That really sounded good!," when said at times other than the practice situation, help make the child feel proud about his communication ability. Because such interactions have been difficult for the child in the past, there can never be too much praise to undo the damage that had been part of past frustrating experiences. Such simple statements as well as acknowledgment that the child is trying, have a significant impact on improving self-esteem.

A system of rewards may be established to encourage the child to work in a cooperative manner and recognize his efforts in working toward improving his speech. Suggestions for designing these systems are offered in Key 18, "Goals, Expectations, Rewards." It is important for the parent to be consistent with whatever system is established to help the child maintain consistency with his newly forming speech habits.

A positive parental attitude regarding stuttering and the child's efforts to improve speech is a valuable requisite for success in speaking. Parents who are so upset by their child's dysfluency that they can't work with him need to change their own attitude. Once the nature of the problem is realized, it is easier to look at the speech problem in a positive way. Parents can then become more active participants in the change process.

Parents are the essential element in a child's learning process. This is especially true in stuttering therapy because it involves not only changing speech behavior, but impacts heavily on self-perception and self-esteem. Your attitude is a significant element in both those aspects of child development.

Part Three

~~~~~~

HELPING THE
STUTTERER AT HOME

When the proper help has been identified and initiated, the next step in the process focuses on the home environment. How to assist the stutterer in developing fluent speech requires the understanding of all those who are part of the child's world—siblings, grandparents, friends, and relatives. In addition, recognizing the relationship of stress, reward systems, discipline, and self-image on the success of learning fluency techniques helps parents provide the support and understanding the child needs to gain the most from the process.

16

~~~~~~

BEHAVIOR: THE STUTTERER AT HOME

T he behavior of the young child who is a stutterer does not differ significantly from that of any normal child. The child passes through the normal stages of growth and development and displays periodic difficulties when trying to express himself. Initially, this communication difficulty is largely unnoticed by the child. In a majority of cases, the dysfluency will pass uneventfully and normal, fluent speech will return.

For the stutterer, the attempts to communicate that are met with stuttering can lead to anxiety and frustration. Physical gestures may be adopted by the child to help release the words. The child may discover that an eye blink will direct attention from the problem and terminate the repetition enabling the word to be produced. The effectiveness of this will eventually wear out and a different method of escaping the inability to talk will be adopted which may be in the form of foot tapping, hair pulling, or word additions to speech.

The frustration of having difficulty speaking may be evidenced in other behaviors that are not associated with communication. Children may anger easily, channeling frustration into more physically aggressive behaviors. They may become combative and argumentative or more physically active and prone to fighting with siblings. This can become aggravated if children become teased about their stuttering at school or in their circle of friends. The makeup of each child is unique and individual; the tolerance and manner in which frustration is demonstrated varies from one child to the next.

It is important to underscore that for the stutterer, fear and anxiety are associated with speaking. The way a child deals with fear and anxiety may affect other behavior in the home. The child may be noted to be more physical in attempts to communicate or in response to communication situations.

The child's behavior is viewed in a social context and how appropriate that behavior is. It is particularly interesting that stuttering may be viewed as a social disease. This does not mean that it develops out of poor social contacts or from inappropriate friendships. It means that stuttering only occurs in a social environment. When the stutterer is alone, he generally does not stutter. It takes one or more individuals for the behavior to occur and the behavior occurs during a communication situation.

Parents can help their child deal with those behaviors that are unrelated to speech but are socially unacceptable (such as physical aggression, situation avoidance) by focusing on the cause of the behavior rather than the negative result. Suggestions for helping the child include dealing with the emotions that are generated by her dysfluency—anxiety, frustration—as well as the emotions created by other people's teasing, criticism, and rejection. If the child can talk about difficult emotions, it is wise for parents to:

1. Praise her for sharing how she feels.
2. Sympathize with the child by relating that it is understood how she is feeling.

3. Suggest and encourage more appropriate behaviors to substitute for those that are presently used when in an emotionally charged situation.

4. Share ways of how they (the parents) have handled similar emotions in other situations.

Communication with the child and among family members is extremely helpful in establishing an accepting environment for the stuttering child. Emphasizing that steps are being taken to help make speech better, reinforcing what is understood about the nature of stuttering, answering questions, and being supportive are the best ways to help control behavior that is inappropriate. Punishment for acting out will not address the cause of the problem and may lead to difficulties in the future as tension and frustration build.

17

PRACTICE

Whether preparing a meal, sewing a dress, learning a golf swing, or playing a musical instrument, practice is essential. The more time invested in rehearsing and practicing, the easier it is to make the new skill become a habit.

Some children understand why they are using their new speaking technique and how it will help them. They will then use it when they sense an approaching block or stutter. But most need to practice before becoming comfortable with this new behavior.

Practice principles are based upon the concepts of learning theory. Some helpful suggestions can make working with the child enjoyable and rewarding. Often, reports of lack of progress or change are the result of failure to follow through with carefully structured practice.

Parents and children always wonder how much time should be devoted to practice. In reality, the more time spent practicing, the faster the new skill will become natural. If a model of the new fluent speech technique is present in a positive, rewarding manner for every waking hour, it becomes a habit more quickly than if it is randomly practiced. This is similar to trying to learn a foreign language. The language becomes quickly assimilated if one moves to the country where he is immersed in it all the time!

Change cannot be expected if only a few minutes a day are sporadically devoted to practice. Practice should be planned for brief periods throughout the day. Several ten-minute periods scattered between breakfast and bedtime, rather than one long session, are most beneficial. Practicing at different times of the day helps the child see the speech technique is not used during special times. The use of the new way of speaking is for all types of situations, during all times of the day.

Short sessions are also better suited to the short attention span of the preschool child. Activities can be quick and varied. Parents who must now focus on the speech technique rather than the message also find it easier to concentrate during the brief sessions. The total amount of time devoted to practice each day will have a direct effect upon learning. In general, the more time spent, the faster the learning curve!

Practice sessions do not require a consistent working area. They can take place anywhere. Practice while cooking, working, car pooling, and so on, allows for more flexibility. Otherwise, finding the time and place for many parents would be impossible. Practice can be portable. Running errands can provide great opportunities for brief yet valuable practice drills.

Opportunities for practice of technique can be included in the child's everyday fun activities. Brief pauses during the course of playing video games can provide the chance to produce sentences or a few answers to questions using the new technique. When watching television together, commercial breaks in programming can afford an opportunity to turn the sound down on the television and allow the child additional time to generate a few sentences to summarize thus far the program he has been watching or answer some questions about unrelated topics. This type of practice helps the child see how his speech is interrelated with daily activities and how it can be used to discuss other subjects of interest such as daily events or interesting games.

It is helpful to maintain a record of practice time and activities. Keeping a calendar that records the time spent each day will not only give a picture of the consistency of the practice but also alert the parent to missed opportunities.

When families plan trips, they often feel this includes a holiday from practice. *There really should be no vacations from practice.* Vacations offer great opportunities to use new speech techniques with unfamiliar people, places, and situations with helpful support and supervision.

Practice can be structured as a game, reducing apprehension and making communicating in real life fun. Praise and reward during the practice sessions as noted earlier accelerates learning and improves chances of success. In summary, practice should be frequent, varied, fun, and rewarding!

One caution should be given regarding practice. If the child in the practice session continues to have difficulty using his speech technique with the task he is working on, it is advisable to discontinue the exercise to avoid frustration. Parents can change to an easier task that has proven successful in the past so the child does not leave the practice time with any negative feelings. The therapist should be alerted to difficulties with the assignment as soon as possible so that the task may be redesigned or you may have improved instruction on how to successfully help your child. Sometimes the assignments may need the guidance of the professional clinician before they are implemented in the home.

18

~~~~~~

GOALS, EXPECTATIONS, REWARDS

T he primary focus for the stutterer is to learn a new way of speaking and to control the stress levels that interfere with fluent speech production. The goal is to learn a new behavior. If sufficient time is invested in practice, progress should be evident. In several of the other Keys, the importance of an award system to accelerate learning has been emphasized. While some may be excited by the process of learning because it is a reward in itself, others require praise and more tangible reinforcement to sustain attention. This is especially true if the change that is to be made is gradual and not readily apparent.

Since periods of dysfluency are usually irregular for the childhood stutterer, sustaining practice during fluent times can be difficult. For the child, as well as many parents, the absence of stuttering is viewed as success and progress. In reality, the fluency may simply be the by-product of decreased stress in the environment and not an indication of any changed behavior. During these stutter-free periods, it is difficult to focus on learning techniques since they are not needed at the time. Therefore, a system is needed that will reinforce as often as possible the use of the new speech technique. The *reward* is predicated upon *use* of the speech technique (much like points are awarded for getting the ball in the basket in the basketball game, not merely shooting at the basket!)

A basic and easy reward system that can be instituted while a child is working with the therapist and parent involves a clean jar and macaroni. The size and the shape of the objects may vary. To begin, a macaroni is placed in the jar for each correct response during the practice time. A predetermined prize will be awarded once the jar is filled. Children, when possible, should assist in the selection of the prize to ensure their interest in the project.

Award prizes within a reasonable time period. It is not good to gain the prize too easily or wait too long to fill the jar. The intent of the reward is to develop a sense of accomplishment. It is most important to learn that doing the correct technique can have a positive outcome. The prize represents the value of the new speaking technique.

During practice, the ultimate goal is to increase the number of correct responses required to obtain a macaroni. Thus, the child must focus longer on the speech technique and less on the prize. Adjusting the size of the jar and/or macaroni is one way to change the size of the prize (e.g., big jar and small macaroni or small jar and big macaroni). Sensitivity to the child's tolerance for frustration as well as her attention span are necessary to keep this method of reward successful.

The first sign that children are motivated is when they initiate practice rather than being directed to do so by the parent. To encourage this spontaneous desire to practice, extra macaroni can be added to the jar for unscheduled, child-initiated practices. Reward can also be given for a cooperative effort during practice. As stated earlier, the learning process should be enjoyable. By encouraging parents to work with their children, extra stress or tension must be avoided for both parties. *Nagging parents are counterproductive to helping children reduce tension and learning.* Making learning a game can be an alternative to confrontation—as long as the child keeps winning!

Prizes may be simple, such as an ice cream cone, a new book, a small car, or delayed bedtime. Some children have worked toward earning larger prizes such as a bicycle (a prize the parents intended to purchase anyway.) This was done in stages rather than as a single reward. For example, a picture of the bike was cut into pieces like a puzzle. Each time the jar was filled, a piece of the puzzle was earned. The end result, over time, was the completion of the puzzle, a new bike, and a new speech pattern!

Playing games during practice and earning a turn after good speech technique is another form of reward. If concentration is poor, a turn can be missed to stimulate the child's attention instead of reprimanding or punishing for lack of cooperation.

In developing reward systems, some advocate what is called negative reinforcement. This is in the form of some type of punishment for not performing the required task. A stronger learning incentive can usually be provided by positive, rather than negative, approaches. There are times, however, when nothing appears to motivate the child. It is at these moments that practice may be tabled and resumed at a later time!

19

~~~~~~

RELAPSE: WHAT TO DO

After you have invested time, energy, and outside resources into helping the child learn a new, fluent speaking technique, and the fluency is consistent, it would seem that the job is done. Indeed, if the process is analogous to learning a foreign language, this would be a reasonable expectation; although sometimes refresher courses are required to sharpen skills not regularly used. This is true, in part, of any new learned fluency technique.

Periodic refresher courses may be necessary to remind the stutterer of the speech principles utilized to maintain fluency. Speech techniques learned in elementary and high school may be disrupted during the college years. Energies during this period of time may be devoted to things such as friends and studies with a shift in priorities from focusing on the development of speech techniques. Many things may restrict the discretionary time available for the stutterer to devote to practice of technique. Reduced attention to newly developed speech skills may result in decreased habit strength and the ability to use fluent techniques automatically. The result may be a return of dysfluency created by the increased stresses related to such things as preparation for graduation or choice of a career. Because the individual has been removed from regular practice for so many years, he may need assistance in recalling the fundamentals of his speech techniques.

There are also other differences associated with stuttering, which do not generally occur with language learning, that may interfere with permanent fluent speech. Apparent regression to old speech habits can be explained in a few ways. It is important to note that stuttering does not redevelop. If it recurs, it is the reflection of the absence of the techniques that manages the stress and reduces muscle tension. Stuttering cannot be cured but it can be kept under control. If the proper fundamentals have been learned at an early age, however, the process of recovery from returned dysfluency is rapid and, more significantly, panic about the new onset of stuttering at this late time in life can be avoided.

Another reason for relapse is inconsistent use of technique. When speech is consistently fluent, the techniques used to reduce stress and muscle tension become less necessary. Fluency generates confidence. Confidence reduces stress. For example, successful, fluent speech in previously difficult situations eliminates the old fear that was once associated with them. As stress decreases, there is less physical disruption of speech and fluency is more consistent. With fluent speech easier to produce, diligence in employing a speech technique lessens and reinforcement of new speech behaviors become reduced. Therefore, when at some point in time stress increases and the need to use techniques becomes essential, the behavior is not as habituated as it should be due to the lack of constant reinforcement. It cannot be called into use automatically. However, when the stutterer reviews the nature and mechanics of speaking techniques to maintain fluency, there is generally a rapid return to fluency and use of technique.

Another form of relapse occurs when the technique is still relatively new. Although the child may be speaking fluently on a consistent basis, stuttering may return when an event causes the stutterer to concentrate on the fear and panic of the moment and then he is unable to focus on anything else. Many well-learned behaviors can seemingly be forgotten during moments of extreme stress. Good swimmers have been reported to drown when overcome by panic created by a sinking ship! In tense situations, focus is on the stressor (the feeling of being out of control) which overshadows the attention that should be placed on what to do under the circumstances (practice learned techniques). Through practice and a gradual increase of tension in the practice exercises, a change of focus can be achieved resulting in the ability to cope and use fluent speech in stressful situations.

The primary cause of relapse is, therefore, the absence of use of speech technique. The cure is renewed practice. This may have to once again begin at the earliest level of learning progressing through increasingly more difficult speaking situations. The process, however, should be quick if the initial learning was soundly based!

If there are frequent periods of relapse, accompanied by high levels of anxiety, counseling should be considered to determine the cause for the individual's inability to maintain the new behavior.

20

PHYSICAL EXERCISE

A s discussed earlier, dysfluency in children is aggravated by stress or tension. One of the best vehicles for reduction of tension and stress is physical exercise. The baby-boomer generation has capitalized on exercise and has incorporated a healthy focus into their life-style. This need is sometimes neglected in children. Since the value of exercise for the reduction of stress has been documented, it is important to consider how it can be formalized in the young child's life—especially in that of the young stutterer.

Parents indicate that their children are overly energetic and that a formal exercise program does not seem to be required since the children already demonstrate a great deal of energy. Many of these children have a difficult time focusing because they are so highly active.

In spite of this, the focus of the child's energy should be examined. Aerobic activity such as running, fast walking, and/or any exercise that increases the heart rate over a sustained period of time has been identified as a stress reducer. Although children may seem to be very active, they often do not engage in this type of exercise program.

Parents should first consult their physician/pediatrician to determine appropriate activities for their child. They may work in conjunction with their speech-language pathologist to determine whether such an outlet would be advantageous to reduce the stress in their child. Many children do not require a formal exercise

76

program to supplement their speech program. However, this avenue should be explored to determine if it would prove beneficial and help speed the process of fluency for the child.

Exercise has been proven to benefit the body in many ways. One beneficial aspect for an individual who is stressed is that exercise can elevate a mood and generally makes an individual feel better. This mood change may be tied to the production of beta-endorphins—brain chemicals—that have been shown to make people feel calmer, happier, and more relaxed. Exercise suggestions for the child that can create increased metabolic rate and potentially reduce stress include the following:

1. Using stairs instead of elevators whenever possible in buildings or in shopping centers
2. Walking to and from school whenever possible (if it is close enough)
3. Walking to see friends who live nearby instead of being driven
4. Riding a bicycle to the store or doing errands while with friends
5. Playing sports with friends as much as possible
6. Reducing sedentary activities such as watching television as much as possible
7. Getting involved in karate or dance classes

21

REST AND RELAXATION

The positive effect of rest and relaxation on stuttering has been documented. Aside from addressing reduction of tension through changing the mechanics of speech production and physical exercise, sometimes it is helpful to focus on how to reduce overall tension in the child. Some stutterers, especially the very young, may not appear to exhibit a great deal of anxiety. Controlling dysfluency may result in an automatic elimination of stress. Other stutterers, especially older ones, develop anxiety prior to speaking events that is increased during the act of speaking. It is in these cases that learning how to control tension and reduce personal stress may be beneficial.

The first step toward assisting in stress reduction is understanding the factors that create stress. Reviewing Key 7, "Children and Tension" will help more carefully evaluate the stress factors in the child's life. Speech is easily produced when the speaker is relaxed, whether the speaker is a stutterer or a nonstutterer. The quavering voice associated with the nervous speaker who must deliver an address in front of a large audience is indicative of the effects of tension in speech production. Researchers have shown that the amount of tension in the muscles of the body as a whole, at any one time, can affect the laryngeal area—the focus of tension for stuttering. When overall body stress is high, the vocal folds show high tension as well. Although it is important for individuals to have adequate tension in their bodies in order to speak normally, abnormally high tension in any speaker, especially the stutterer, can have negative consequences.

Helping the young stutterer to reduce tension can be accomplished through a variety of methods. The first is to ensure that the child receives adequate rest. Bedtimes should provide ample opportunity for sleep since the absence of adequate sleep has been identified as a stressor. Established systems and routines such as consistent bedtime, bath time, opportunities to watch television or read, and so forth, help control anxiety in the child and may serve to eliminate some stress.

Examine mealtimes and establish a noncompetitive environment for conversation. When there is an understanding among all of the siblings of the rules governing conversation during these times, a certain level of relaxation can be obtained by eliminating competition for attention.

For the very young child, it is difficult to develop formal relaxation techniques. Suggestions focus primarily on developing parent awareness of how to reduce home tensions and support the fluency. Under the guidance of a therapist, relaxation exercises of a formal nature may be attempted with the child. Some of these can be tried at home and done jointly by the child and parent. For example:

> Consciously create tension in the speech muscles (clench teeth and tighten the jaw on command) and then release that tension and attempt to be as relaxed as possible. Also focus on clenching the fist, counting to ten, and relaxing the fist; or

tightening the toes and relaxing them. Using these body parts, it is easy to see if the child is able to follow directions. This can help to begin an understanding of how he can make muscles tense and then relax them.

Ask the child to speak as quickly and loudly as possible. Then instruct the child to speak as softly and slowly as possible. This provides a contrast between the tension required for the first task and the relaxation that is found in the second. Varying between these tasks a number of times can help a child tune in to how he is physically producing speech. It will also help him to understand what it may feel like when he is under stress, and then how it feels when he is more relaxed.

While sitting quietly, help the child draw a picture either on paper or with their imagination of a scene they feel to be quiet and restful. Talk about the picture and how it feels to be in this relaxed space. Encourage them to remember this feeling (and picture) when they find themselves in a difficult speaking situation.

Another process used to help cope with the tension is called desensitization. In this process, a child is presented with speaking situations that are gradually more stressful. For example, a child may practice new speech techniques first with people who are aware of the child's training, such as the therapist and parents, and then increasingly with people who are unfamiliar with the child's training, such as a friend, then several friends, then with the teacher, then in front of the class, and so on. The child is assisted through the easier tasks and given positive reinforcement so that he gradually may accept increasingly more difficult and stressful challenges. A level of calmness must be maintained during the speaking task to be able to be successful.

In general, observing the child's diet, setting limitations and routines for family activities, and working with the therapist to develop exercises to enhance relaxation are all positive steps toward reducing stress and improving fluency for the child. An understanding of the importance of relaxation is also valuable for the child so that he may replicate and utilize the techniques learned when he is away from the guidance of the home or school environment.

22

~~~~~~

COPING WITH BROTHERS AND SISTERS

C hildren who stutter often have brothers and sisters who are fluent. If the stutterer is the oldest child in the family, parents may be concerned about the speech and communication of their other children.

When the stutterer is surrounded by other more verbal children, there is great competition for parents' attention. The communication process becomes very competitive with many ideas being expressed from different individuals simultaneously. Dinner table discussions can be quite active with each child discussing events of the day and interrupting others' conversations. For the stutterer, this can be a very stressful situation. The desire to maintain the same speaking speed as their brothers and sisters can create the final stress that can trigger the stuttering.

Under such circumstances, it is recommended that parents develop "turn taking" discussions where each child is given the opportunity to present her thoughts while the others courteously await their own turns. This reduces the competitive aspects of communication, and serves to reduce stress as discussed in Key 21, "Rest and Relaxation."

If the child is in therapy, it is advisable to share this information with the siblings. They, too, can be part of the homework process and work along with the parents to help establish the new speech behaviors. This involvement can serve to improve their understanding of the problem of stuttering and increase their tolerance during dysfluent moments.

Siblings can often accompany the parents to the therapy sessions to participate or observe. This experience makes them part of the solution to the problem. Their encouragement and support will foster reduced anxiety and potentially improve the child's competence level and self-esteem by this acceptance from others. The involvement of the family helps the child become more comfortable with using her new speech technique since it becomes an accepted part of daily life by all those around her. Caution should be exercised, however, in inviting others to therapy. Sometimes the child regards this time as special and may feel that others are trespassing on her private space.

Tension may increase if an overbearing sibling who is already rivaling for attention begins to chastise and correct the young stutterer who is not using newly learned speech skills. It is important to achieve a balance between helping the child versus correcting her.

One child had great fun competing with his sister to see who could catch the other not using the learned speech technique—while only one really stuttered. The sense of a game removed the task from being a speech exercise and transformed it into a fun activity that continually rein-forced learning.

Playing board games as a family can present addition-al opportunities to include the brothers and sisters into practice. The stutterer can be encouraged to ask siblings questions or answer their questions in between each move or play of the game. This places the competition away from the speech exercise and places it in a more socially acceptable game context. This type of opportunity, however, enables the child to become more comfortable using a different way of speaking with those at home.

When parents are busy or have difficulty working with their child, cooperative brothers and sisters can often be the solution to ensuring that sufficient time can be devoted to practice. In Key 15, "How Parents Can Help the Stuttering Child," the importance of this is discussed. With the help of other family members, the learning process can be fun and more easily made a way of life for the child.

Brothers and sisters can help provide opportunities for the child to rehearse her speech technique outside formal practice. They can accompany the child to fast food restaurants or observe her buying tickets to a movie while encouraging the use of the speech technique in these more difficult situations. These situations help to increase reinforcement of the newly learned skills in real-life situations with positive reinforcement and support from individuals with whom the child feels safe and secure. These are all opportunities to help develop confidence in the child which, in turn, improves fluency.

23

~~~~~~

COPING AS PARENTS

Parents basically feel that they are, in some ways, or entirely, the cause of their child's stuttering. This sense of guilt cannot escape being conveyed, in some measure, to the child and results in heightening anxiety for him. It is important to analyze behaviors to determine how much parents are really contributing to the problem.

Since stuttering has been defined as a physical response that is triggered by tension, tension-producing factors are important to identify. People react to tension in a variety of ways. The stutterer, however, exhibits one of the most overt and obvious reactions—dysfluent speech.

Tension-provoking factors have been discussed in Key 7, "Children and Tension." Review these to begin an inventory of areas that may be contributing to unnecessary stress. As this is done, be careful to note areas that may be stressful but are a necessary aspect of child rearing and, thus, cannot be changed. Necessary but stressful events may include established rules for bedtime or cleaning up after themselves; punishment given for improper behavior; or unpleasant situations such as visiting the doctor or dentist. All of these things are essential parts of a child's life and cannot be discarded because they are judged to be stress-producing.

Analyze the manner of discipline. If too many rules are set or there seems to be excessive discipline, reassess the effectiveness of the current system and determine less stressful ways of achieving the desired outcome. Psychologists report that overly constrictive limits can make a child feel hostile, anxious, or fearful. Most of us follow reasonable standards and guidelines for discipline and rule-setting. These should not be abandoned in the mistaken assumption that they may be creating too much stress and contributing to the stuttering. Good parenting prepares children for their future and helps to shape values. After all, in adulthood they will have to abide by the laws and rules of society and assume responsibilities.

The stutterer, although affected by stress, will also have to cope in this world of rules and regulations. The best and easiest place to learn how to function and communicate is within a home environment that replicates the values the child will encounter when he enters school and, later, the work world. Consequently, it is advised not to alter parental standards to make home unnaturally comfortable in a mistaken effort to reduce the stress level. Psychologists believe that children who learn rules and regulations usually feel more secure. Established parameters reduce uncertainty which in itself is a cause of stress. Thus, what may be viewed as authoritarian and stressful (i.e., rules and discipline), actually serves to be beneficial emotionally and psychologically in later years.

Parents are not the cause of their child's stuttering. Although some literature on the subject has stated that children stutter to gain their parents' attention or imitate behavior of another family member, these ideas have proven to be untrue. It is the child's reaction to stress—good and bad—that is the trigger for the dysfluent speech.

Parents should be cautious in setting unrealistic demands or putting too much pressure to achieve on their children. If these demands are beyond the ability level of the child, they may be causes for undue stress. These factors should be carefully examined and adjusted to be more appropriate for each individual.

Additional aspects for parents to consider include:

1. Show interest in what the child is saying and give him full attention when he is speaking to you.
2. If the child appears to be hurrying to talk, let him know that there is time to listen and there is no need for him to rush.
3. If you are involved in a project while the child is trying to gain your attention, acknowledge that he is speaking to you but request that he waits until the project is finished so that he may have the attention desired.
4. Do not label the stuttering behavior as "bad." Acknowledge that he is having difficulty and that he will have to overcome it.
5. Be prepared to counsel and help the child if he reports instances of being teased or made fun of at school by his peers. Be supportive and understanding. Reinforce that the practice he is doing and the therapy he is receiving will help him to cope better with the problem.

24

COPING WITH FRIENDS AND RELATIVES

T he people most willing to offer advice about how to correct a child's speech usually are friends and relatives. These are the people who have encouraged parents to seek help despite advice from the family pediatrician. Unfortunately, often these individuals do not understand the nature of the problem and, although well meaning, may not be able to offer helpful advice on how to handle stuttering.

After gaining knowledge about the nature and treatment of stuttering, it is important to share this with other significant family members and friends. It is also helpful to alert them as to what is being done to help the child. Those that can be helpful in the process include the spouse, siblings, grandparents, uncles, aunts, and cousins. In addition, those friends that are close to the family and child should also be educated.

Parents often carry tremendous guilt from the constant remarks from well-meaning relatives about how they must be the source of the stuttering and how, because of their child rearing practices, the child may be scarred for life. It is important to help others understand the true nature of the problem. This serves as a positive resource for others as well as a way for the parents to alleviate some of their own anxiety about the problem.

Including all these individuals in the therapy process can have the following results:

1. Relieve pressure on the parents, permitting them to focus on helping their child
2. Help others understand the technique the child is learning in therapy so that they can also provide reinforcement and opportunities for practice
3. Create a comfort level for the child and opportunities for using her new technique; the more people involved, the better. The child becomes more comfortable because the new speaking technique is commonly used and accepted and not reserved simply for practice times with the parents.

Perhaps the most important role friends and family can play is to serve as a source of positive reinforcement for the child. Rather than showing concern, they can offer praise on how great the child's speech sounds. They should not be overly demonstrative. Simple recognition is enough to help establish a positive self-image and a feeling of accomplishment.

One helpful technique is for the older stutterer who understands the processes she is involved in to explain to others what she has learned and what she is doing to improve her speech. This process, called *education and demonstration*, is educational and beneficial for both the listener and the stutterer. Stutterers usually demonstrate initial resistance to the task because they do not relish calling attention to their speech, although they will acknowledge that they realize others are aware of their dysfluency. Stutterers can do this for family as well as schoolmates. The listener benefits by learning more about the process and understanding more about stuttering. This leads to better acceptance and more patience when confronting individuals who have speech disorders.

The benefit to the stutterer is a continual reduction in anxiety level when approaching feared speaking situations. The stutterer most often perceives the listener to be threatening. This mental image is usually overly exaggerated. The listener is often far more uncomfortable than the stutterer. Once the stutterer begins to approach others and discuss the problem of stuttering, a better understanding of how she is perceived develops. A more positive self-image can develop and the stutterer can gain confidence during the process. Apprehension can be replaced with confidence as more people become educated by the stutterer. Soon, fear of situations also can be decreased because the negative reaction that was anticipated and heightened the stress is now replaced with more concrete expectations of positive behavior and acceptance.

When this process begins at an early age, children can avoid the negative experiences that are the result of misperceptions and erroneous, preconceived ideas. By including others in their therapy process, the new speaking behaviors are felt to be more natural.

25

SELF-IMAGE

W hile working on the mechanics of improving speech and fluency, it is important not to neglect the psychological/emotional side of the child. Psychologists agree that a good self-image is the single most important tool for successfully facing the problems, issues, and crises that arise in everyday life. It is the key to the way a child will treat himself and be treated by others. Even the youngest of children can suffer diminished self-esteem or self-image from experiences related to their stuttering. The often sudden onset of dysfluency is very unsettling to the child. One parent related how she felt that her son was not called upon by the teachers in school. In truth, he simply refrained from speaking because he was fearful of stuttering and was unable to give the answers.

With misconceptions like this one prevalent in society, it is not difficult to understand why a child can develop a poor self-image. Young children are usually not thought of as mature enough to be focusing on the world and a sense of how they are perceived. Children can readily understand, however, the concepts of "stupid"..."unintelligent" ..."slow"..."different." These labels have meaning for them, and, although they may not possess the sophistication to fully comprehend their implications, they do absorb negative images about themselves.

Children of a variety of ages can present themselves with feelings of hopelessness because of their communication difficulty. Since speech is a primary component of most professional and social interactions, these children view their future as dim. Yet with proper intervention, this perspective can be changed.

Self-image is learned. Every time a child is criticized, rejected, teased, hated, or ignored, there is a negative effect upon his feelings about himself. Many of these things occur for the stuttering child because of his communication difficulty. By the same token, self-image can be made better through praise, acceptance, love, and attention.

Capitalizing on the use of a new fluent speaking technique, parents should encourage the child to verbalize successes experienced when using the new technique. These may be minor at first, outweighed by stuttering episodes. But it is helpful if the parent can focus the child on positive experiences such as using the technique to answer a question in class or order something at a fast-food restaurant. By recognizing the use of a new technique in situations apart from practice times, the child is helped to understand that a new behavior can be learned and that the potential to be successfully fluent exists. This helps the child to look at his future in a more positive way.

Psychologists have determined that the messages that people give themselves can become self-fulfilling prophecies. For example, when a child tells himself that he is unable to hit a baseball or talk on the telephone, this eventually becomes the reality. The stress that gets created by the fear of entering into the situation can make success in that endeavor impossible. The same is true for speaking and fluency. If the child tells himself that he can't succeed or can't change his speech, there becomes little reason to doubt these assumptions. This ultimately can eliminate motivation to make any changes because the situation appears to be hopeless.

The power of positive thought has been explored and found to be a strong antidote to the hopelessness created by negative beliefs. The field of sports psychology focuses on working with teams to build the positive concept of winning before entering the playing field. From ice skaters to football teams, successes have been documented based on the improved confidence level of approaching the task with a sense of winning. The same is true for the stutterer. The belief that fluency is possible helps perpetuate better speech as well as reduce stress levels. When stress is reduced, the cycle of improved fluency can begin. As confidence builds, and positive thoughts are reinforced, fluency becomes a reality.

The following principles are valuable in helping your child improve self-image:

1. *Positive reinforcement.* Praise for doing something creates an incentive to repeat the activity again. Praise may be verbal ("I'm so proud") or tangible (a trip to the zoo, an ice cream cone).

2. *Repetition.* Learning to feel good about oneself can be accomplished through many repetitions of the reinforcement and the positive ideas presented.

3. *Time.* Learning takes place for individuals at their own pace. Give the child time to master the task with reinforcement throughout the project.

4. *Focus.* Self-esteem can be enhanced by focusing on effort and achievement and downplaying failures.

5. *Criticism.* To help a child improve how he feels about himself, criticism should be avoided. Rather than criticize an action, tell the child what to do that would be better.

6. *Compliments.* Give the child several compliments each day in many different areas but be concrete

and specific. ("You really sound terrific. Your new speech technique is great.")

7. *Environment.* Create an emotionally supportive household environment; express confidence in the child's ability; express pleasure at being the child's parent; treat the child with respect.

The most difficult thing for parents in helping children develop a better self-image is addressing their own behavior and restructuring how they communicate with their child. It is helpful to examine how able the parent is in accepting compliments and criticism himself before he can assist the child in these areas. Both parent and child need to understand that it is acceptable to make mistakes and learn how to use them as a learning experience. If these areas can be focused on in a positive way, then the child will be able to feel better about himself. As this confidence grows, stress level should be reduced and the child will begin a positive approach to life with greater fluency.

26

HEREDITY

From a research perspective, it is difficult to conclude with 100 percent certainty that stuttering is inherited. However, in studies of identical twins, one of the best ways to observe identical biological subjects, a 77 percent occurrence of stuttering in both twins has been found. Only one out of three fraternal twins of stutterers also stutters. This seems to point toward a genetic link since the biological structure of fraternal twins is parallel, not identical, and the occurrence of dysfluency is reduced.

Children of stutterers are more likely to stutter even if their parents stopped stuttering long before they were born. In addition, an increased occurrence of dysfluency is found if a relative stutters or once had trouble with her speech but reportedly has outgrown it. The roots of a problem can be found beyond the limits of the immediate family. An early warning sign that the dysfluency observed in the young child may not be simply a developmental stage is, therefore, a confirmed family history of stuttering.

27

DISCIPLINE

P arents often feel or are advised that if their child is beginning to stutter, they should reduce the stress and tension in the home. One aspect that gains immediate scrutiny is the method of disciplining the child. Discipline obviously is a stressful enterprise for both parent and child.

Discipline can begin for a child as young as six months old, according to psychologists. Rules are set and attempted to be followed in an effort to help the infant to live happily and comfortably with the parents. This is accomplished through rule-setting.

Psychologists urge that parents understand that discipline doesn't essentially mean punishment. Rather it is viewed as helping children to make parental standards their own. If limits need to be set, children cannot do it on their own and need guidance.

It is often evident that children misbehave just to get attention. It is beneficial to try to make this unnecessary by giving them lots of good, positive attention. This will improve self-image as well as decrease instances of unnecessary dysfluency.

A beneficial suggestion for parents when they encounter a great deal of stress in disciplining their children is to establish a *time out*. Psychologists report that it works well for both the parent and child. Sometimes this can be accomplished by sending the child to a corner, to his room, to a designated chair, or sometimes the parent can remove herself from the situation. This avoids prolonged arguments and confrontations and can sometimes help alleviate stress.

Parents should not avoid disciplining their child since creating a home environment that is stress-free is not adequate preparation for what will be encountered in the real world. It is important to help the child understand limitations and deal with his fluency in a variety of stressful environments which includes unpleasant situations in the home that require being disciplined.

28

STRESS

F actors that add stress serve to increase dysfluency for the stutterer. Life events and change are primary stress factors. Often these are beyond control and cannot be avoided. There are many stressful events, or traumas, that can adversely affect the fluency of the stuttering child. In all these situations, it is important to note that it is not the event itself that causes the stuttering, it is rather the tension generated by the individual in response to this event that causes the stuttering to occur.

Trauma

Parents usually exhibit a great deal of anxiety when they discuss traumatic events that have affected their child. They feel responsible in some way for allowing these events to occur and harm their child. It is often easier for them to attribute the development of the stuttering to an actual event. People often seek a cause-and-effect relationship when trying to solve a problem. By doing this, it is less difficult to handle, especially when the problem is unfamiliar and difficult to understand. This is the case with stuttering.

There are many life events that can create stress and aggravate the problem of stuttering. These include the birth of a new baby; a parent returning to work; the hospitalization of the child or close family member; the loss of a family member through death; or any other situation that creates uncertainty and change. These events can be either the trigger for the first evidence of stuttering, or they can be the factors that aggravate an already dysfluent speaking pattern.

Patience and understanding and extra attention focused on the child during these difficult periods can help to alleviate some of the stress associated with them. While usually this is a stressful time for both parent and child, displaying extra patience and understanding should prevent any lasting effects once this period has passed. Increases in stuttering at such times should not be viewed with alarm. Increasing the frequency of practice, as well as offering extra praise for effort that is demonstrated to use the new speaking technique, will serve to at least maintain the learning that has thus far occurred. Once the stresses have passed, it should be easier for the child to focus on practice and use of speaking technique.

Divorce

Divorce is a major life event signaling change for all family members and can be especially stressful for the children. Child specialists have felt that it may be the "emotional divorce" preceding the legal divorce that harms the child more than the divorce itself. Many lives can be shattered during the process of divorce.

During the process, parents themselves are under extreme stress and feel quite unlike themselves. It is difficult to expect the child to be able to cope any better than the parent may be. Suggestions from psychologists indicate that if the child is old enough, she should be included in discussions about the unhappiness that is being experienced by both parents.

The child will be most influenced by the way the parents conduct themselves during this time. The calmer the atmosphere, the better the chance that the child will feel less threatened. All children should be helped through this difficult time regardless of their age. Current theory tends to indicate that there is no critical point in child development when a divorce might be "easier." Therefore, calm and communication can be invaluable to minimize the child's stress through this period. However, fluency may be adversely affected as a result of the stresses that will be present.

Aside from the divorce itself, changes in living arrangements will also bring with them new stresses. Stress is created not only by the immediate absence of a parent and family fragmentation but also by changes in routine and living style. While parents experience the same stresses (and more) during this transition period, they can try to help their child understand that stress reactions to these types of things are normal. Acknowledging that speech may be a little more difficult for the stutterer during this time can help ease anxiety until fluency levels improve as everyone adjusts to the new living situation.

Anticipatory Stress

The common tensions that are associated with normal life events as well as the physical tension created by speaking can also be compounded by what is called *anticipation of an event* or *anticipatory stress*. Anticipatory stress is learned and, as the name implies, builds in anticipation of the feared event. Such tension develops out of the remembrance of the stuttering that occurred in a particular situation or with a certain individual. The situation can be confused as the source of the stuttering when, in reality, it is merely the setting in which the stuttering occurred. If the stuttering recurs in the same type of circumstance, the individual begins to approach the event with increased apprehension and tension. The individual learns that it was associated with the unpleasantness of stuttering. Not wanting to repeat such painful experiences, stress can build in anticipation of having to participate in a similar event or situation.

In addition to situations such as speaking in class or talking to relatives, people or events may also clearly be identified as stress-provoking. Stutterers may also develop a fear of certain sounds or words. When asked, stutterers will report that they can't say "hard sounds like t or d" or their names without getting stuck. Parents indicate that the child will always get stuck on "p, b, d." Again these become confused as the source of the stuttering when they were merely what was being said when the tension reached its peak to create the repetition or speech block.

The stress created by anticipation is very real. The best analogy as to what happens is as follows: If someone is riding a horse and it throws her, she would probably get up, dust herself off, then remount. She might be a bit more apprehensive than before the fall, but that would soon pass if nothing further occurred. However, if the same horse threw her five times, she would probably never want to see the animal again. In fact, passing the stall where it was kept would be stressful! If the horse's owner showed her a burr that was under the horse's saddle that caused the behavior, it would probably still take some time and many positive experiences riding the animal to increase the comfort level, if she was even willing to try again!

In this scenario, the rider learns to be afraid of the animal because of the negative events associated with it. The easy assumption was that the animal was at fault rather than an outside factor (the burr) that created the behavior in the horse. Even when this is identified, it takes some time to feel confident again and unlearn the negative experiences.

The same is true for the child or adult stutterer and sounds, words, and events that have been associated with negative dysfluent experiences. For these individuals, a speech technique alone may not be sufficient to decrease the vocal cord tension. Sometimes relaxation and other speech techniques may be required to reduce that anticipatory stress. When the individual realizes that the fear is learned and can, with diligence, be unlearned, the new technique should be sufficient to maintain future fluent speech.

In the majority of young children, the problem of anticipatory stress is usually not too great. In general, these children by virtue of their age, have had limited opportunities to reinforce to any significant degree events that provoke stuttering. Those children who can name persons, places, words, or sounds that they know they "can't say," require the use of further stress-reducing techniques to relax tension levels. The parents' role in this process is invaluable in maintaining appropriate levels of relaxation as well as identifying sources of stress.

Parents should understand that stress is instrumental in creating dysfluency in the stuttering child. Avoiding unnecessary pressure and understanding situations that can evoke stress help to enable the child to cope better with her speech difficulties. The parents can help the child identify these situations and understand them. Using newly learned speech techniques and those concepts explored in Key 21, "Rest and Relaxation," provides a unified approach in helping the young stutterer become fluent.

Part Four

HELPING THE
STUTTERER AT
SCHOOL

A significant portion of a child's time for nine months of the year is spent in school. It is crucial to include this environment and all those that are part of it in the fluency learning process. This section addresses the stutterer and his concerns in school. It discusses young preschool children and follows their needs through kindergarten and elementary school to the more complicated teenage years. Children with special learning considerations are also addressed.

29

THE SCHOOL SPEECH-LANGUAGE PATHOLOGIST

C hildren of all ages from preschool to high school have access to the services of the school district speech-language pathologist if a communication problem is present. Within school systems in most states, the services of a speech-language pathologist are available free of charge for children who exhibit speech, language, voice, and/or fluency disorders. The laws in each state vary regarding services that are mandated free of charge. Some states provide assistance in private schools as well as in public schools. Others may restrict coverage to certain treatments. Questions regarding the availability of speech therapy services should be directed to the local school district in the Department of Special Services. Consult the phone book and call the local Board of Education to request the Office of Special Services, or speak with the principal of the school closest to home.

If information is not available through these sources, you may contact the State Department of Education located in the state capital for availability of services.

Public Law 94-142 addresses the rights of individuals with speech disorders and the availability of services for them. Clarification regarding how an individual state is implementing this law should be addressed to the State Department of Education, Division of Special Services. Additional resources may be obtained by contacting the American Speech-Language and Hearing Association in Washington D.C. The Consumer Helpline is 1-800-638-8255.

School speech therapists face many obstacles in attempting to implement a therapy program. Generally the biggest difficulty is the lack of parental involvement. Once the child enters a school program, parents often abdicate all responsibility for the treatment process, relying on the school to solve the problem. The nature of fluency therapy necessitates a total, daily commitment to learning the new speech technique as well as developing confidence and a positive attitude in the child. Parents should meet or speak with the therapist at least weekly to determine home practice goals and problem solve situations that appear to be difficult for the child. Homework is essential for establishing the correct habits.

The school speech therapist's time is sometimes limited because other school functions (assemblies, special programs, and so on) take priority over allotted speech therapy appointments. School vacations and holidays further reduce available opportunities to work on fluency. The size of the caseload of the therapist also places limitations on what can be offered to the child. Often school speech therapists must see 70 to 100 children per week. These are some reasons why the home program must remain an integral component of treatment.

Before enrolling in the school therapy program, parents should explore the therapist's background in stuttering treatment to ensure that the time being spent taken from regular school work will be productive. As with any therapy program, it is helpful to have clearly defined goals, proposed timelines for their completion, and progress measurements during the process. Children enrolled in school programs are generally given an Individual Educational Plan (IEP) which defines the goals and timelines for the year. These should be clearly understood and reviewed by the parent with the therapist not only at the start of the program but also frequently during therapy to ensure that the child is progressing.

The assistance of school therapists in stuttering therapy affords many advantages. They have the opportunity to control a large segment of the child's daily speaking environment and vary the stress that is present. They can regulate the level of difficulty at which speech techniques can be practiced. Their presence can reinforce the proper techniques and offer support during speaking situations that the child may judge to be difficult. From chatting with the janitor to asking the principal questions to answering the school phone, the child can rehearse his new speaking technique with the support and guidance of a knowledgeable professional.

The therapist can also serve as a liaison to the classroom teacher. In this role, the therapist acts as a resource for both teacher and class, and can assist the child in educating and demonstrating his new speech technique to the class to further reduce stress. Numerous opportunities to encourage the child to use technique outside the structure of the therapy setting are at the disposal of the school therapist. For example, seeing the child in the lunch room, bus line, or at recess and asking a simple question so the child can rehearse his fluent speaking technique at unexpected moments is good reinforcement. Such encounters can foster spontaneity in the speech technique and assist in the development of a new automatic speech behavior.

The best success can be achieved by using a team to help the child learn his new speaking skill. The more team members who reinforce the desired behavior, the easier it becomes for the child to remember what is expected. The new speech behavior becomes more natural and a normal part of the daily routine when several people are supporting the learning process.

30

∿∿

CLASSROOM TEACHER

A side from parents, one of the most influential people in a young child's life is the elementary classroom teacher. The significant amount of time children spend with their teachers daily and the role teachers fill as educators and guides in the learning process gives them a great deal of responsibility for those in their care. This time is often when the child is most impressionable and open to learning. The teacher, therefore, is a powerful player in helping the child develop and perfect her new fluent speaking techniques.

One parent indicated that her son's first grade teacher refrained from overly encouraging the child to read out loud for fear of placing undue stress upon him. She indicated she thought he probably stuttered when he was silently reading and didn't want to aggravate his stuttering problem. The result was that, once the parents discovered this misconception, the school year was already at an end and the child had fallen below his expected reading level. A summer tutor with a better understanding of stuttering was hired to make up the lost learning. This is a clear demonstration of how a lack of understanding of the problem of stuttering had a negative outcome for the child.

In addition to this child's lost opportunities, the broader picture should be viewed. This was but one of the hundreds of children who would ultimately be influenced by the ideas of this teacher. Without proper education, this misconception could be perpetuated and others could also suffer. In addition, many other students could have their views on stuttering shaped by this erroneous concept and, in the future, unfairly judge stutterers based upon it.

It is essential to provide the public—especially educators—with the correct information about stuttering. Increasing knowledge about the problem is important for developing the best environment for fluent speech. By using new speech techniques, stutterers are the best ambassadors for changing perceptions about the disorder, especially when they discuss the problem and its treatment. It is, therefore, critical that the teacher be a key part of the process of improving the child's use of the speech technique by reinforcing its use in the classroom.

The speech-language pathologist in the school will serve as a resource for the teacher and assist the parent in understanding what the disorder stuttering is and how the child can be helped. The concept of the team continues to include the parents as a vital link between the school services and the home setting.

If the child has experienced success and is fluent following intervention, then the school therapist and the classroom teacher can enhance and reinforce the skills that were learned in therapy supporting the carryover process. Now instead of being excluded or given special considerations regarding speaking tasks in school that may create stress, the child should be encouraged to participate in all class activities. She may need additional support to help develop the confidence that she is able to accomplish these tasks. Avoiding the task will not give her confidence in her fluency. If the speaking technique is newly learned, the introduction of verbal classroom activities (such as doing oral book reports, reading aloud, and giving speeches) should be gradual and preceded by rehearsal with the therapist or a parent to ensure success. As confidence builds, preparation may be reduced and speech more spontaneous.

If a private therapist has been initially engaged to help the child, she should try to be available to visit the school and offer support to the child as well as provide education for all staff involved in the learning environment. It is recommended that teachers coordinate their activities with the school therapist to ease transition and ensure the most comprehensive program for the child.

31

BEHAVIOR AT SCHOOL

D uring the early school years, stuttering children are accepted by their peers and the dysfluency may go unnoticed. As they become older, they may become the subject of teasing. Children with strong self-images may not feel the sting that such criticism can create. Most children, however, react by becoming upset and withdrawn. They prefer silence in school and in most situations that require talking rather than attempting to speak.

As with the young stutterer in the home, the stuttering child in school can become disruptive and act out physically because of the frustration created by his difficulty in communicating. It is reported that children may spend a great deal of time in detention or the principal's office because they become physically aggressive and fight with those who tease them. These children become labeled as "troublemakers"and "difficult to manage." In reality, it is the frustration created by an inability to express themselves that is channeled into aggressive behaviors.

Again, as with the younger child, being supportive and understanding is critical to help them through this difficult period of time. This alone, however, will not suffice. It is important that there be intervention in the school and communication with the classroom teacher as well as school administrators to help them understand the problem and the child's behavior. If the child is in therapy, the child and his therapist can educate the teacher (and any other school personnel) on the realities of stuttering—its possible causes, its treatment, and the emotional effect on the stutterer. This can be part of the structured therapy session and is an integral part of a successful therapy program.

If the behavior problem continues to exist with few changes in fluency, additional assistance may be required to help the child deal with his frustration and anger. This may be the time when inclusion of the school psychologist as part of the team may be wise. The concept of a team approach is important. The parents as well as the teacher, school therapist, and psychologist are essential members of the team. There should be a clear understanding of each person's role in the process and communication among all team members should be frequent.

The child must learn that socially unacceptable behaviors will not be tolerated. More positive outlets for frustration should be developed until the communication skill improves to the level where minimal difficulty exists and the child is better able to express himself. Attention should be addressed to the sources of the child's anxiety which may be creating negative feelings about himself. For example, the experience of listeners reacting negatively to the stutterer's attempts to speak, failed self-improvement of speech, and/or failed success in previous therapy can frustrate and depress the stutterer. The inability to succeed and overcome the problem also contributes to low self-esteem and self-concept. All these factors should be considered when trying to assist the child.

32

~~~~~~

PEER PRESSURE

H umans are intrinsically social animals. From the youngest toddler who enjoys being with children her own age to the gregarious teenager whose life seems to center around friends, interaction with others is a very important part of life. For the young stutterer, speech difficulty can have a significant impact on social interactions.

Stuttering is viewed as a socially damaging disorder. One's speech is a major element in how people form opinions and judgments about one another. The inability to communicate clearly and effortlessly may create a judgment of impaired sociability or lower intelligence.

Young toddlers interact briefly with other children but generally go about their own business. They are empathetic to others and try to comfort someone who may be upset. They are primarily focused on motor activities and play, paying no attention to others' speech.

As children enter preschool, they become more interactive. Although taking turns is difficult in many activities, they are able to share. Four-year-olds love to play with other children and can be verbally assertive. Here, dysfluency can hinder the normal assertiveness of the child and begin to create frustrations.

As conversation skills develop and evolve throughout the preschool and kindergarten years, communication difficulties have a greater impact. Dysfluency may be unnoticed by close friends, but in the young school-age years when children seek attention, and are competitive, it may set them apart from kids who notice this difference and generate teasing from them. Friends of the child may be protective, but depending upon how well developed the young stutterer's self-image is, the response may be upsetting and increase tension.

During adolescence, although peers play a very important part in a child's life, researchers have shown that parents and peers are not opposing forces during this time. Children more readily listen to their parents on questions relating to important issues. It is the time when parents can be supportive of the child by listening to any frustrations she may be encountering and offering positive directions to help. While peers may tease the stuttering teenager, parents can be supportive and offer direction in how to improve the problem.

For the stutterer, peer pressure may be exhibited in a nontraditional sense. Rather than trying to make the child conform to a behavior because others are doing it, the pressure may be from peers in the form of ridicule or criticism. Parents can help their child through this period by assisting the adolescent in discovering strengths and special talents contributing to positive self-image. The importance of this is discussed in Key 25, "Self-Image." At this point in development, it is critical to focus on the internal view the child has of herself. Even though her communication disability inhibits her during this time of intense peer interaction, feeling good about herself can lessen some of the pain associated with this difficulty.

It is helpful to increase the frequency of speech practices with the child and try to anticipate situations in which the stress may be high. Assist the child in learning how to anticipate difficult situations and plan how to communicate and handle herself in them. It also helps to encourage the adolescent to form friendships with peers who share the same beliefs that she does and support her. This can create the positive environment to develop confidence and enhance the environment for the development of successful speaking techniques.

33

~~~~~~

TODDLERS AND PRESCHOOLERS

C hild psychologists describe toddlers as individuals trying to learn how to master and perfect their environment. During this period of development, children have an increased desire to imitate adults. They seek a great deal of approval and delight in pleasing their parents, their most important audience. The child at this age is described as "loving the world and eager to learn from it."

Toddlers begin to develop self-assertion and a drive for independence. These are aspects of growing self-esteem. At this time, due to the increased environmental exploration and social interaction, parents need to set clear limits to help children learn appropriate social behaviors. Doing so comes in direct conflict with the toddler's growing need for self-assertion.

During this time, there is a great desire for the young stutterer, as well as the normally fluent child, to communicate to parents all of the new experiences they are encountering. Unfortunately, the complexity of language and the stress that evolves in trying to put thoughts into words can increase the stress and further disrupt fluent speech.

In addition to the stresses that are created in trying to express ideas, other anxiety is present at this point in development. This is the time that fears of things that previously never seemed to concern the child, develop. He is frightened by loud noises such as dogs barking, vacuum cleaners, or lawn mowers; or fearful of animals; or objects. Although the fears seem unreasonable to the parent, they are very real for the child and create a great deal of stress.

At this point, the first stages of sibling rivalry develop. It has been described as a "fierce and deep jealousy and hatred of the other children in the family, particularly the younger ones." These negative feelings can create stress in the child, especially if the stutterer is at the receiving end of an older sibling who demonstrates them. All of these situations can create more stress and increase dysfluency.

Parents should communicate any of these observed problems and developmental behaviors to the child's teachers at school. It helps to alert those in the school environment to the child's increased stress. Preschool teachers can be helpful with assisting the child to better understand some of these anxieties. In addition, they can help reinforce the speaking techniques in a potentially less stressful environment than the home. They can support the parents' efforts to help their child improve his ability to communicate during this increasingly stressful period in his life.

Parents sometimes say that their child's speaking becomes more dysfluent when he is in preschool, or it increased when he began to go to preschool. They question whether the child should remain at home and not be placed in this stressful environment. It is possible that no matter how careful the selection process was, the school may not be right for the child. If the child appears to be unhappy and resists going to school in the morning, it is recommended that parents speak with the child and determine if he can express what he is feeling. It may be beneficial to sit in the classroom and observe as well as talk with the teacher. Most teachers are willing to assist parents in determining what the actual problem is and help the family through the transition period. If these suggestions do not prove successful and the child continues to be unhappy about going to school, and becomes increasingly dysfluent, it may be wise to reconsider sending him and instead wait for him to become more mature. It is important to note that the increase in dysfluency is not a direct result of the school environment. It is merely a reflection of increased stress and tension in the child and may be an indicator that there is a problem although he is not able to verbalize exactly what it is.

The best solution to increased dysfluency during this period of time is to investigate potential causes of increased stress, increase communication with the child and others that are working with the child, and continue to practice speech techniques that will improve fluency.

34

~~~~~~

KINDERGARTEN AND ELEMENTARY SCHOOL

While many children in today's society attend preschool programs, for some the first introduction to the educational system occurs in kindergarten. The formal educational system in this country is structured such that children enter the system between the ages of four-and-a-half to six years. The entrance of the child is predicated on the *readiness* for a formal learning situation—good physical health; emotional readiness to separate from the parents; and the ability to interact with adults and children who are unfamiliar.

The introduction into the school setting creates many changes for young children. Schedule changes begin to occur in the routines that are familiar to them. They are now required to follow schedules and established patterns in the classroom leaving less time for free choice. Many more rules are placed upon them regarding behavior and conduct. In this setting, verbalization becomes more important. The ability to communicate ideas and thoughts become one measure of assessing the child's capabilities and mastery of what has been taught.

In addition, the number of social contacts significantly increases. From the level of the child's own peer group to the number of authority figures that are present (including teachers, school staff, and the principal), the social context expands, and with it, the stress environment. The transition began with play and moves to real work. With this transition comes additional stress.

Some children who previously were not identified as stuttering begin to exhibit their first dysfluencies in this environment. This may be the parents' initial awareness that there may be a problem. This is because the child's tension level had remained below the point of triggering the muscle tension to create the stuttering. The addition of all of these stressors and changes in routine created the environment that raised the physical level of tension to a point to set off the dysfluency.

If parents notice a change in their child's speech behavior, it is recommended that they speak with the classroom teacher to determine if the same dysfluency is present in the classroom. Consultation with the school speech therapist, if one is available, is also suggested. At this time, parents should ask about the type of approach the therapist would use and further information regarding stuttering. In addition, the team that will assist the child throughout her school years now begins to form.

It is important that the classroom teacher be included throughout the elementary school period in the speech treatment process. Since it is recognized that stuttering cannot be cured (only controlled), it is essential that the techniques learned become incorporated into all life situations. As stated before, communication on a regular basis among the individuals involved in the child's education is essential to ensure the child's achievement, positive peer interaction, and the subsequent development of self-esteem.

Careful selection of understanding and supportive classroom teachers throughout this educational experience are important for the stuttering child. The child should never be given the impression that she is "different." The shaping of this concept weighs heavily in the hands of the teacher—the person the child is with the majority of the day. In addition, this is the individual who directs the attitudes and ideas of all of the peers who are part of the stutterer's environment.

As discussed earlier, one of the difficulties for improving fluency for the school-aged child is motivation. Parents must work closely with school personnel to ensure proper motivation and determine techniques that they can utilize to enhance and encourage this in their child. The stuttering child is required sometimes to spend extra time away from things she enjoys to work on her fluency techniques. Finding this time can become difficult as the child progresses through the elementary school years. Often, stutterers may be labeled as "different" because they must be taken out of class to see the speech teacher. Parents should be sensitive to the child's feelings about this. If the child's attitude begins to deteriorate and she becomes unhappy and reluctant to take extra time away from her friends and studies, parents should meet with school personnel to discuss alternate approaches.

If the child has been in speech classes for many years, and progress is minimal, a "vacation" from speech may be advisable. During this time, the current program should be re-examined and alternatives planned. Sometimes learning can be enhanced when a period of rest is given.

35

~~~~~~

TEENAGERS

A dolescence is a time for which few parents are totally prepared. Adolescence signals a period of rapid growth and change. Some of the changes are biological, some intellectual, some emotional, and some social. All of these changes, complicated by the communication difficulties of the stutterer, can make the role of parenting even more challenging.

It is important to recognize that the transition from elementary school to middle or junior school and then high school can create temporary disorientation for the child. Self-esteem can falter and feelings of alienation and vulnerability may arise. This shift is created by the organizational changes in the educational process from elementary school to middle school to high school.

In elementary school, children have a single teacher who knows them personally; children are rewarded for trying hard; they are supervised all day; and they are familiar with the structure and demands that are placed upon them. By the time they enter a new high school environment, the shift is to many more authority figures evidenced through a variety of teachers for different subjects, performance-based grades, independence, and more freedom.

A child who has attained a certain level of fluency and ability to control his speech in the elementary environment may suddenly experience a significant increase in dysfluency. Parents often become frustrated and concerned. Unfortunately, they often blame the child for failing to pay attention and becoming lazy with his speech. In reality, it is the shift in stresses and attention that have made the ability to incorporate newly developing speaking techniques into everyday life more difficult.

The best method to approach this change process is to increase communication with the child. Patience is required to help during this transition process. It is helpful for the child to have parental support and understanding rather than criticism while he is undergoing these new experiences.

It may also be difficult for parents during this time to accept that the child no longer looks to them for the answers to all of his questions. The shift toward independence makes it more difficult for parents to establish the guidelines that may be required for children to learn the new speech behavior.

Parents may contact the therapist for the child's school and meet to discuss the previous therapy program and the child's progress and responsiveness. Exploring the options available in this new setting for improving speech are important to determining and planning for continuation or maintenance of the new fluent speech skills.

In this setting, the child should be an integral part of the planning process for his speech program. During elementary school, activities to improve life-style or behavior could be structured and the child could be required to participate. Once reaching adolescence, *encouragement* rather than *requirement* must be the direction of parental assistance. Teenagers must recognize the need to change their speech behavior. Their motivation and cooperation in the process is essential for success. This can become frustrating for parents who stand by and see the teen struggling in attempts to communicate while they are powerless to assist and correct the problem. During this time, offering guidance, understanding, information, and support are the only tools available to the parents.

On a positive note, motivated teenagers may make great strides in a fluency therapy program because they are motivated to change. The process of improving stuttering is a learning task that is accelerated by motivation. During this time, teenagers may also realize the value of relaxation, exercise, and proper diet in helping reduce stress, enabling them to maintain better control of their fluency.

The parents may not be included in the home assignments as they had been in the past. Being available to their child to assist him with his assignments may prove beneficial if the stutterer seeks help from them. Goal setting and a reward system are appropriate for teenagers as well as younger children. The type of reward, however, will change and may take the form of an extension of bedtime, watching programs they like on television, going to a concert, or getting posters for their room.

The period of adolescence is difficult for parents and teenagers. Changes occur on many different levels and there is no clear road map through the process. A great deal of uncertainty is present each day. Parents often have difficulty letting go and allowing their children to exercise their independence. This is particularly true when they know that there is a problem that needs to be addressed. Teenagers must shift into the role of being responsible for their speech rather than having parents be their directors. Parents need to assist their child in making this transition and assuming this responsibility. During the process, patience, understanding, and acceptance are the most successful ways to bridge the change.

36

WHAT STUTTERERS SAY BOTHERS THEM MOST

Stutterers focus on themselves and their speech problem and often have an incorrect perception of how the listener perceives them. Most stutterers feel ashamed by their speech and assume that they are judged by those to whom they are speaking. They fail to realize the discomfort of the listener.

Listener discomfort or uneasiness is expressed in many ways that can be more stressful, rather than helpful, to the stutterer. A primary complaint of stutterers is the impatience of the listener. This impatience serves to imply the need for the stutterer to speak more quickly. Impatience can be reflected in interrupting the stutterer when she is trying to speak but is in the middle of a block—and the interruption provides no positive result. Rather it only serves to increase the tension level. The result of trying to speed up speech results in a decrease in ability to speak at all due to the tension required to perform more quickly.

Often, in an attempt to make talking easier, the listener will finish the sentence for the stutterer or supply missing words. Unfortunately, these words may not reflect the intent of the speaker. Thus, there is increased frustration for the stutterer who must try to correct the incorrect message that has been created for her by another.

In some cases when the stutterer is having difficulty, those with her will speak for her. Sometimes this provides a measure of relief for the stutterer and an escape. Most often, however, as the individual gets older, this creates more damage to self-esteem and self-image because the stutterer appears to be unable to do something that is normal and natural for everyone. They perceive themselves as failures and may withdraw even more from social interactions and communication.

In addition to these elements, other issues to avoid with stutterers include criticism for not practicing frequently enough or using their new techniques; placing them in speaking situations and making them talk when they are uncomfortable; and placing them unprepared into new social situations, especially when people will be present and they are expected to be sociable.

In the early stages of developing a new speaking technique, parents' assistance in making special allowances for certain school activities is desirable. Allowances may include, for example, being excused from making oral book reports, participating in school assemblies, or other activities that may call attention to the child and her speech. These situations should not be totally eliminated but may be modified so the child can feel success rather than anxiety when she participates. As the child grows older, these arrangements may not be desirable. As she improves in her ability to communicate and utilize fluent speech techniques in more complicated conversational situations, she should be encouraged to participate. Adequate preparation and rehearsal before the activity itself may serve to increase confidence and improve success.

37

~~~~~~

CHILDREN WITH SPECIAL NEEDS

S ome children may have additional problems with learning or behavior that may complicate the fluency therapy process. This may include children with learning disabilities, attention deficit disorders, hyperactivity, or those who evidence some degree of mental retardation. In most cases, these children can be taught to improve their fluency and modify their stuttering with minor adaptations to the teaching program.

Special-needs children require modifications in the teaching process for most aspects of their learning. In fluency teaching, the major program difference is that it becomes slower and there is a great deal of repetition of tasks to develop the required speech behaviors. Rather than rely on the child to recognize the opportunity to self-initiate the new speaking techniques outside of therapy, these children need to learn the speech technique so that it becomes almost automatic and replaces the usual speech pattern. To make any behavior automatic requires mass amounts of repetition, practice, and rehearsal. Because of the extent of the practice required, goal attainment and movement to new targets and tasks will be slower. However, in these special cases, once a goal has been mastered, it generally becomes relatively permanent and habituated.

Perhaps most importantly with these children, the reward system is an essential ingredient of the treatment program. Most learning is difficult for these children. With their learning difficulty has come frustration and failure. Because of this, praise and reward can make the children feel more positive about themselves and their ability to learn. As with all children, these factors are part of self-image and self-esteem which, when raised, can lower overall stress through increased confidence. This new attitude can have an automatic positive effect on fluency.

With special-needs children, the most important element is patience. The learning process may be slower, but if carefully structured, progress should be steady. Spontaneity of technique usage may be less evident but reminders to use technique should produce the desired new fluent speech behavior.

Part Five

~~~~~~

HELP FOR THE PARENT

T his concluding section presents information regarding additional resources available to parents of stutterers. Private therapy is explored as an alternative treatment source if the other options discussed are not appropriate or available. It is recognized that parents often need support themselves during the course of their child's fluency program to avoid the frustration that can develop during the learning process. The role of the family and support groups in helping parents to maintain their energy throughout this time is discussed.

38

~~~~~~

FAMILY

P arents are most often the first to identify a problem with their child. When a difficulty is determined, whether a learning disability or speech dysfluency, the process of seeking help can be very draining on the parent. Searching out the appropriate resources, investigating the quality of what is available, and then following through with the child are all emotionally and physically draining for the parents. Providing the child with the support, understanding, and patience that are required during the change process also requires a great deal of energy from the parents.

The family is the most vital resource that the parents have to replenish their energy supply. The same support and understanding given to the child can also be invaluable when given to the parents by those whom they love. All members of the immediate and extended family including grandparents, aunts, uncles, and cousins can participate in the process of helping the child improve.

Parents need to communicate to these significant others all aspects of the child's communication problem and its treatment. These individuals can assist the parent in practice and reinforce what is learned in therapy. By understanding the situation, criticism in child management can be reduced.

Encouraging family members to be patient with the child when they are trying to communicate can alleviate some of the stress of the speaking situation. An understanding of the treatment process and the probable causes of stuttering, may help change the expectations of the family and make it easier for them to relate to the stuttering child. By expressing quiet understanding and listening, family members can provide support for the child and encourage her willingness to communicate. This behavior provides support not only for the stutterer but also for the parents and is important in successful resolution of the difficulty.

Since stuttering will not go away and is not curable, it is important that those involved with the child and parent understand so that they can be part of the change and improvement process. It is a lack of understanding that fosters criticism when potential relapse occurs or when speech behaviors become increasingly dysfluent. Since these periods of time are particularly difficult for the parent, additional stress is not productive. Rather, the oasis that can be provided to the parent by an understanding family can ease the tensions that are present and enable the parent to offer more to their child.

39

~~~~~~

PROFESSIONALS: PRIVATE THERAPY

When children are enrolled in school therapy programs, parents generally assume that the problems are being addressed and that additional resources are unnecessary. Unfortunately, this is not always true. The following danger signs should alert parents to the potential need for additional outside intervention.

- Therapist reluctance to include parents in the process
- Unavailability of therapist for parent conferences
- Lack of speech homework and home exercises
- Absence of any visible progress and improvement over a period of time
- The need for fluency therapy over a period of several years with minimal improvement
- The absence of goals and monitoring of goal attainment
- Use of generic treatment plans or Individual Educational Plans (IEP) that are not modified to reflect the child's needs or progress
- Large group (4–5 children) therapy sessions where there is only one stutterer and the rest have other speech and/or language problems
- Therapy scheduled only once a week for a short period of time or in a large group
- Therapist's lack of experience with any stutterers

- Therapist's inability to explain the nature of the problem and rationale for the approach used to both child and parent
- Limited time available for the stutterer due to caseload demands

These reasons are obvious cause for parental concern and would warrant seeking outside, more experienced help. In addition, if the child appears to become uncooperative and refuses to willingly work with home assignments, a private therapist may be necessary to intervene and motivate the child. Sometimes only a brief consultation or a few sessions may be sufficient to set up a program that can then be implemented by the parents and the school clinicians.

The private therapist may also work with the school therapist and the parents to train them in techniques that will be successful with the child. Some private therapists may be a considerable distance from the family and school. The specialist, however, can be a resource for others who are more readily available to work regularly with the child (such as the school therapist).

When distance is a concern, progress can be monitored through the use of audio or videocassettes. While these do not replace the necessary one-to-one contact essential for quality treatment, they can serve as valuable supplements between sessions so program modifications or alternate exercises can be implemented in a timely manner. Periodic consultations by the parents and/or school therapist with this stuttering specialist are valuable to review progress and modify treatment goals. The treatment results can be most rewarding when all individuals associated with the child, both at home and school, are willing to learn, follow therapy directives, and maintain active communication regarding progress.

40

~~~~~~

SUPPORT GROUPS

S tuttering tends to be a very isolating problem and people are reticent to talk about it. They are reluctant to acknowledge the behavior when speaking to a stutterer. Stutterers sometimes rarely come in contact with other stutterers. They view their problem as unique and hidden. Parents have been counseled that it is a developmental stage and will be outgrown. When this doesn't happen, they often feel guilty in having not addressed the problem. As discussed earlier, there are many emotional aspects to the problem of stuttering.

Over time, the benefit of support groups has been proven—especially for chronic problems. Both parents and child benefit from such groups. It is here that they become aware that they are not alone and that others share similar experiences. In this environment, techniques for fluency can be reinforced and information can be exchanged on how to cope in difficult communication situations.

Unfortunately, few groups exist that meet this need. Some therapists have developed groups for parents and clients so that they may meet on a regular basis and exchange helpful information. When a child is enrolled in a therapy program, it is beneficial to investigate whether such a program exists. Parents can request that the school therapist or private therapist arrange a meeting of parents and patients. If this is not feasible, parents may request the names of other clients from the therapist, to form such a support body. Children who stutter report positive experiences from such meetings. They realize that they are not alone and that others have similar problems. Some of the mystique is removed from the fluency difficulty. They often realize that they are not abnormal since others do share the same handicap. When they meet adults with successful careers who are stutterers, a more positive focus on their future is created. Motivation for change and improvement is also stimulated.

For further information about stuttering and/or other speech disorders, the best resource is the American Speech-Language-Hearing Association. The Consumer Hotline (1-800-638-8255) will be willing to supply information regarding communication and its disorders. The American Speech-Language-Hearing Association (ASHA) is located at 10801 Rockville Pike, Rockville, Maryland, 20852.

QUESTIONS AND ANSWERS

What is stuttering?

Stuttering is the word used to describe the repetition of sounds or words that disrupt the normal, fluid flow of speech.

What causes stuttering?

Stuttering is caused by a combination of factors. Although the exact cause remains uncertain, experts agree that the disrupted speech is the result of a physiological breakdown of the vocal mechanism that is triggered by stress.

Why do some people stutter when they are tense or nervous and not others?

All individuals are unique and react to stress or tension in different ways. The physical makeup of people also varies. Because of this uniqueness and variability, stress affects people differently. All people have an internal, physical stress point that reacts to the tension first. In stutterers, this stress point is the vocal cords. In others it may be the stomach, head, back, and so on. When the vocal cords become too tense, they spasm and stuttering occurs.

Is stuttering hereditary?

Although no genetic evidence presently exists that stuttering is hereditary, research has shown that stuttering, as well as other stress-related disorders, tends to run in families.

Is stuttering caused by a traumatic experience?

While a traumatic experience or stressful event may be the first evidence of stuttered speech, the event in itself is not the cause of the stuttering. It may be one of the factors that triggers the physiological reaction to create the disturbance in fluent speech. The tension associated with the event may simply have been so great that it triggered the combination of physiological events to cause the dysfluency of speech.

How can my preschool child be feeling so much stress when I have tried to keep my home as comfortable and relaxed as possible?

It is important to note that the muscle tension that creates stuttering is not simply related to negative factors that are commonly associated with stress. When a child is excited or happy, the muscle tension present may be equivalent to that of when he is nervous or upset. Stuttering can occur during happy times such as going to a birthday party or a special event as easily as it can be evidenced during more negative situations such as when he is being punished. The physical creation of tension is the same whether it is excitement or nervousness.

How do I get rid of the secondary characteristics of stuttering such as eye blinking or foot tapping?

In successful treatment programs, the elimination of the dysfluency by introduction of a new speaking technique will automatically eliminate these secondary characteristics. It is believed that they are often the reflection of the tension and struggle. Once that tension and struggle is eliminated, they too are eliminated.

Should I decrease disciplining my child to make our home less stressful to avoid stuttering?

Children need to learn standards of behavior to be successful adults. If punishment is excessive and extreme, it should be reviewed and revised. However, stuttering children need to be able to be fluent in stressful situations as well as in those that are comfortable and relaxing. It is therefore not advisable to reduce the standards within the home that are similar to those they must meet when they are outside of that environment such as in school and later in life in work situations. Disciplining your child is an important aspect of child rearing and should not be eliminated simply because the child stutters.

What should I tell my child to say to the children at school who make fun of his speech?

If the child has been working in a program to improve his speech, he may take this opportunity when others make fun of him to thank them for the reminder and begin to use technique. If the child has developed a healthy attitude about why he has difficulty, it is easier to face the thoughtless behavior of others. When stutterers lack confidence or have low self-esteem, it is difficult to respond well in such situations. This is a difficult question to answer because of the uniqueness of each individual and his response to criticism and teasing. Knowing your child and how he responds in these situations, you must tailor your guidance to what you feel would be the best way to respond.

Will my child outgrow his stuttering?

Because the nature of the problem is the result of a physical focus of tension in a specific place in the body, and this tension focus rarely changes with maturation, the problem is generally not outgrown. In some cases, where the stuttering is part of the normal speech development process, the potential is greater that the dysfluent speech will pass.

Can stuttering be cured?

With continued research in the field of stuttering, the remediation of the disorder is hopeful. At the present time, with the current level of understanding of the problem, stuttering can be controlled but it can not be cured. The control, however, can be maintained and afford easy, normal communication.

How old should my child be before he can get help?

Children as young as two-and-a-half years of age can be helped to develop better speech habits. Other beneficiaries of early intervention are the parents. They can learn more about the problem before misconceptions can develop. Education and understanding are important to reduce anxiety and provide the most benefit to the child.

What is the prognosis for the future for my stuttering child?

If an understanding of the problem is provided early in life and skills are learned to avoid the stuttering behavior, future frustration and anxiety about communication can be avoided. A healthy approach to stuttering can prevent the development of behaviors that could make the stuttering more severe.

What should I tell the rest of the family about my child's stuttering?

Once you understand the cause of the problem, share the information with the family. Helping them learn more about the problem will enable them to assist you and the child in correcting it!

What factors can be controlled to help contribute to reduce stuttering?

Stuttering can be reduced if stress-creating factors are low. However, it may return once they are increased (as generally happens in the natural course of life). External variables that can contribute to stress should be monitored, such as the intake of sugar, chocolate, caffeine, as well as some food additives. Aerobic exercise is a good way to reduce the overall stress level which will indirectly help decrease dysfluency.

Does fatigue or illness have any effect on stuttering?

These two variables have major impact on fluency. When tired or ill, the body is not functioning as efficiently as normal. It has been observed that stuttering commonly appears to increase under these two conditions. When they are resolved, speech fluency improves.

Can I work with my child to improve his speech or do I need professional help?

If the problem is in its early stages, parents can often successfully help their child. Seeking information from a trained professional and working with the child and therapist can have a major impact on improving fluency. If the child refuses to work with the parent or a more intense stress is apparent, professional help is essential to create the proper treatment program. The parents, however, must be a part of whatever course of treatment is prescribed.

How long should therapy take?

Because learning aptitude is highly individual, it is difficult to generalize a concise time for the course of treatment. The treatment plan should be available and progress charted so that improvement is continual. The amount of practice outside the therapy setting will also determine the length of the process.

How often and how long should I practice with my child?

Since the answer to controlling stuttering is learning a new way of speaking, and since learning requires practice, the more frequent the practice, the faster the goal will be achieved.

Once the technique is learned, should practice stop?

Because the techniques employed to maintain fluency are learned and not the natural behavior of most individuals with whom we communicate, the newly learned speaking skill will receive little reinforcement in the everyday world. It is easy for habits to become weak in such an environment. Just as athletes who excel in sports continu-

141

ally practice to sharpen and strengthen their skills, so, too, should stutterers maintain some form of daily practice to ensure their fluency technique.

If my child is speaking to me and stuttering, should I stop and correct her?

Until a new behavior is learned (and understood) that replaces the normal dysfluent speaking pattern, stopping your child could prove very frustrating. Unless she really knows how to fix the problem, she will not be able to make a permanent change. Without the skill of a habituated technique to assist her, she will need to be stopped continually because she is most likely unable to control her stuttering. The best advice is if your child becomes stuck and unable to speak or she repeats sounds or words and is aware of this, let her know you see that she is having difficulty and that you will help.

How can I help another family member or friend who stutters?

To help others, share with them information about the cause of the problem. Be supportive of their efforts to improve their speech. Remember that the daily maintenance of fluency for most stutterers is not easy and requires vigilance and continual self-monitoring. Encourage them to seek help even if they have tried in the past. Present advances in treatment are proving far more successful than past therapy programs.

What should I do when I am speaking to someone who stutters? Should I help him finish his words?

A majority of stutterers that I have interviewed feel that quiet patience on the part of the listener is most helpful to them when they are having difficulty. They don't like others to finish their words and thoughts. Although it is difficult for the stutterer and uncomfortable for the listener, the behavior of choice is patient listening.

If my pediatrician tells me that my child will outgrow the problem, should I wait?

If your child appears to be experiencing great difficulty when trying to speak, if he reverts to pointing instead of speaking, if he appears frustrated, then seeking professional assistance is advised. Be cautious about your selection of a consultant. Be sure she is credentialed to work with communication problems, is knowledgeable about stuttering, and is willing to include you in all aspects of treatment. Even if the child is not included in formal therapy, an informational session for yourself may be invaluable in preparing for any future treatment needs as well as giving you constructive advice on ways to assist your child during this dysfluent period.

What should I tell my child's classroom teacher?

The most important thing to do is *educate*. Just as you would instruct family and friends in what you have learned about the nature of stuttering, include the teacher in the process. When your child is beginning to learn her technique, she may not be able to employ it successfully in all required school speaking situations. As your child's proficiency (and confidence) grows, more demanding speaking assignments (oral reports, class presentations) can be introduced. Enlist the help of the teacher in this process to maximize your child's success.

GLOSSARY

Anticipatory stress the learned stress reaction that increases muscle tension in response to feared events, situations, or people.

Avoidance behaviors techniques adopted to abort stuttering including word substitutions, use of nonverbal communication, or withdrawal from potentially stressful speaking opportunities.

Babbling the stage in the development of speech where the infant produces the sounds of the language in an effortless, easy manner.

Block the moment in disruption of speech where the vocal cord tension reaches a threshold that creates a disruption in the rhythmic movement. Term used by stutterers to describe the inability to continue speaking.

Dysfluency (disfluency) term used to describe the disruption in the normal flow and rhythm of speech. Also may be used to describe stuttering or stammering.

Fluency continuous forward flowing movement evidenced in speech by the movement from sound to sound in a non-disruptive manner demonstrated by effortlessness.

Larynx (voice box) physical structure in the throat in which the vocal cords are located.

Normal dysfluency period in speech development between the ages of two and five years characterized by effortless repetitions of words.

Self-esteem an individual's perception and value of self.

Spasm the reaction of a muscle to stress causing an involuntary contraction rendering it incapable of further movement.

Speech-Language Pathologist (therapist, clinician) an individual specially trained in the area of communication and its disorders.

Stammering disruption in the fluid rhythm of speech; also may be called *stuttering*.

Stress in medical terms, the body's reaction to events or individuals that are judged to be threatening, which includes, but is not limited to, an increased level of tension in muscles. Muscle stress is also created by physical movement or activity. The term is conventionally used to describe the causes of the reaction as well as the reaction itself.

Stressors events, situations, people that lead to stress.

Struggle behaviors inappropriate gestures or facial expressions that accompany stuttering.

Stuttering term often used to describe the disruption in the normal fluid rhythm of speech. This may be the term applied by a listener who perceives this disruption in speech. May be identified as sound or word repetitions or prolongations.

Tension muscle tightness. Also used to describe psychological or emotional state.

Tension threshold the point of maximum tolerated tightness of a muscle. Beyond this level a muscle will spasm.

Uncertainty stress the stress triggered by anything that happens for the first time or which is difficult to understand.

Vocal cords (vocal folds) muscles in the larynx that, when vibrating, provide the source of sound for speech production.

RESOURCES

American Psychiatric Association, *Childhood Disorders*. Washington, D.C.: Author, 1988.

Ames, L. B., *Questions Parents Ask: Straight Answers*. New York: Clarkson N. Potter, 1988.

Brazelton, R., *Toddlers and Parents: Declaration of Independence*. New York: Dell Publishing, 1989.

Conture, E., *Stuttering*. Englewood Cliffs, New Jersey: Prentice-Hall, 1990.

Dell, C., *Treating the School Age Stutterer: A Guide for Clinicians*. Memphis: Speech Foundation of America, 1979.

Dodson, F., and Alexander, A., *Your Child: Birth to Age Six*. New York: Simon & Schuster, 1986.

Eisenson, J., *Stuttering: A Symposium*. New York: Harper & Row, 1958.

Epstein, L., and Squires, S., *The Stoplight Diet for Children*. Boston: Little, Brown, 1988.

Fraser, J., and Perkins, W., *Do You Stutter: A Guide for Teens*. Memphis: Speech Foundation of America, 1987.

Fraser, M., *Therapy for Stutterers*. Memphis: Speech Foundation of America, 1974.

Fraser, M., *Stuttering: An Integration of Contemporary Theories*. Memphis: Speech Foundation of America, 1980.

Ham, R., *Therapy of Stuttering: Preschool Through Adolescence*. Englewood Cliffs, New Jersey: Prentice-Hall, 1990.

Heins, M., and Seiden, A., *Child Care: Parent Care*. Garden City: Doubleday, 1987.

Hegde, M., *Introduction to Communicative Disorders*. Austin, Texas: Pro Ed, 1991.

Leach, P., *Your Baby and Child: From Birth to Age Five*. New York: Alfred A. Knopf, 1990.

Leith, W., *Handbook of Stuttering Therapy for the School Clinician*. San Diego: College-Hill Press, 1984.

Logan, R. J., *The Three Dimensions of Stuttering*. Austin: Pro-Ed, 1991.

Peines, M., *Contemporary Approaches in Stuttering Therapy*. Boston: Little, Brown, 1984.

Peters, T., and Guitar, B., *Stuttering: An Integrated Approach to its Nature and Treatment*. Baltimore: Williams and Wilkins, 1991.

Phillips, D. with Berstein, F., *How to Give Your Child A Great Self-Image*. New York: Random House, 1989.

Steinberg, L., and Levine, A., *You and Your Adolescent: A Parent's Guide for Ages 10–20*. New York: Harper & Row, 1990.

Schwartz, M., *Stuttering Solved*. Philadelphia: J. B. Lippincott Co., 1976.

Schwartz, M., *Stutter No More*. New York: Simon & Schuster, 1991.

Selmar, J. W., *Help! My Child is Starting to Stutter*. Danville: Interstate Printers and Publishers, Inc., 1989.

Selmar, J. W., *Help! The Child is Stuttering*. Austin: Pro-Ed, 1991.

Trace, R., "*Stuttering: Early Intervention is the Key to Successful Treatment*," *Advance* 2:9, May 1992.

Wall, M. J., and Myers, F. L., *Clinical Management of Childhood Stuttering*. Austin: Pro-Ed, 1984.

Wells, B., *Stuttering Treatment: A Comprehensive Clinical Guide*. Englewood Cliffs, New Jersey: Prentice-Hall, 1987.

INDEX

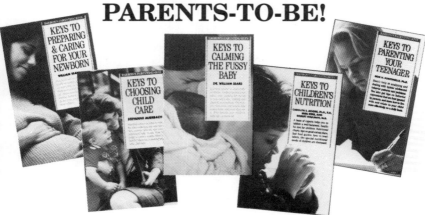